Key Concepts in Mental Health

Recent volumes include:

Key Concepts in Social Research
Geoff Payne and Judy Payne

Fifty Key Concepts in Gender Studies
Jane Pilcher and Imelda Whelehan

Key Concepts in Medical Sociology
Jonathan Gabe, Mike Bury and Mary Ann Elston

Forthcoming titles include:

Key Concepts in Leisure Studies
David Harris

Key Concepts in Critical Social Theory
Nick Crossley

Key Concepts in Urban Studies
Mark Gottdiener and Leslie Budd

The SAGE Key Concepts series provides students with accessible and authoritative knowledge of the essential topics in a variety of disciplines. Cross-referenced throughout, the format encourages critical evaluation through understanding. Written by experienced and respected academics, the books are indispensable study aids and guides to comprehension.

DAVID PILGRIM

Key Concepts in Mental Health

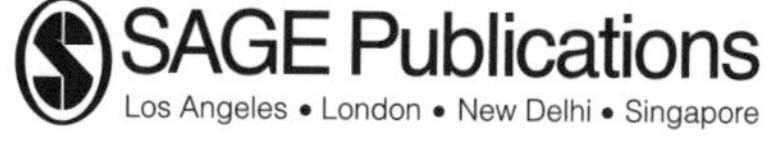

First published 2005

Reprinted 2005, 2006, 2007

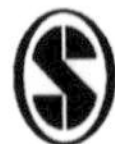

SAGE Publications Ltd
1 Oliver's Yard
55 City Road
London EC1Y 1SP

SAGE Publications Inc
2455 Teller Road
Thousand Oaks, California 91320

SAGE Publications India Pvt Ltd
B 1/I 1 Mohan Cooperative Industrial Area
Mathura Road, New Delhi 110 044
India

SAGE Publications Asia-Pacific Pte Ltd
33 Pekin Street #02-01
Far East Square
Singapore 048763

British Library Cataloguing in Publication data

A catalogue record for this book is
available from the British Library

ISBN 978-1-4129-0776-7
ISBN 978-1-4129-0777-4 (pbk)

Library of Congress Control Number: 2004116567

Typeset by M Rules
Printed in Great Britain by The Cromwell Press Ltd, Trowbridge, Wiltshire

contents

PART 3 MENTAL HEALTH AND SOCIETY

acknowledgements

Writing a book of this sort, with its broad remit and pressure to condense, inevitably has involved capturing and distilling ideas, information and knowledge claims from many sources. This has entailed crossing the boundaries of several disciplines (mainly social history, health economics, comparative religion, philosophy, psychology, psychiatry, sociology and social policy).

The challenge was eased by my work with and influence from a number of friends, teachers and colleagues over a number of years including: Judy Allsop, Don Bannister, Bill Barnes, Richard Bentall, Pat Bracken, Peter Campbell, Mick Carpenter, Katherine Cheshire, David Denney, Leslie Hearnshaw, Linda Gask, Norman Ginsburg, Pat Guinan, Nigel Goldie, Ray Holland, Eric Karas, Ron Lacey, Richard Marshall, John Martin, Shula Ramon, Phil Salmon, John Shotter, David Smail, Geraldine Strathdee, Phil Thomas, Andy Treacher, Lesley Waldron and Fiona Williams. Discussions with these people, as well as their published work, have undoubtedly shaped the way I have addressed the task set by this book.

I would like to thank Nigel Rogers and Steven Pilgrim for their views on the draft entry about creativity. Finally, particular thanks are given to my wife and long-term collaborator Anne Rogers. Her recent competing professorial duties meant that (unusually) she does not appear as a co-author this time round. All of the entries in the book contain her influence and help.

David Pilgrim, October 2004

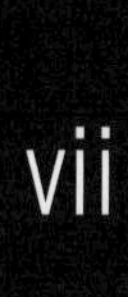

author's preface

The form of this book resembles most of the others in the *Key Concepts* series produced by SAGE. I have written 50 entries of two types. One or the other is determined in style by the breadth of the topic being considered. In the first, I have summarized the topic with no citations in the text and simply provided a further reading list at the end. The second type of entry is a traditional short essay, with references given in the conventional way in the text. The reference section at the end is intended then to double up as a further reading list.

The book is divided into three parts. The first explores the contested nature of *mental health and mental health problems*. Probably most psychiatrists (and some clinical psychologists) writing this book would have simply provided a reduced and diluted version of a psychiatric textbook in this section. However, I have opted to provide traditional psychiatric descriptions but also rehearsed criticisms of them. This means that I may be having my cake and eating it. However, my hope is that it will enable readers to consider both claims from within, and criticisms of, professional knowledge. I have also addressed topics like pleasure and creativity, which are less visible in the mainstream clinical literature produced by psychologists and psychiatrists.

In the second part, the focus is on *mental health services*. This provides several accounts of the ways in which mental health work is organized and the professional interests involved in service delivery. It also addresses the role of 'users and carers' in relation to modern mental health services in developed countries.

The third and longest part addresses a range of topics related to *mental health and society*. This builds on discussions in the first part, with its emphasis on the contested nature of mental health. Mental health work occurs in a social context. It has a particular social history and it has been fraught with political and ethical controversy. This part tries to capture this picture.

Each entry starts with some key summary points to orientate the reader, and a definition. With the occasional exception, I have constructed each definition afresh. As a consequence, they reflect my views of the topic in hand. I have endeavoured to strike a balance between description and critical analysis in the entries but I am aware that the former, as well as the latter, reflect my knowledge and values. These will have shaped what I have omitted, what I have included and how I have chosen to discuss each topic.

PART 1

Mental Health and Mental Health Problems

Mental Health

Definition: Mental health is used positively to indicate a state of psychological well being, negatively to indicate its opposite (as in 'mental health problems') or euphemistically to indicate facilities used by, or imposed upon, people with mental health problems (as in 'mental health services').

Key points: *• Three different uses of the phrase 'mental health' are examined • Reasons for the use of 'mental health' in preference to other terms, such as 'mental illness', are discussed.*

Alternative connotations of the term 'mental health' indicated in the above opening definition will be discussed below, in relation to positive mental health, mental health services and mental health problems.

- *'Mental health' as a positive state of psychological well-being* A sense of well-being is considered to be part of health according to the World Health Organization, which in 1951 described it as 'the capacity of the individual to form harmonious relations with others and to participate in or contribute constructively to, changes in his social or physical environment . . .' (World Health Organization, 1951: 4). This has been built on over time (see entry on mental health promotion). Various attempts have been made to describe mental health positively by psychoanalysts (Kubie, 1954) and social psychologists (Jahoda, 1958). The latter reviewer described the term 'mental health' as being 'vague, elusive and ambiguous'. The range of definitions offered can be challenged on a number of grounds, related to their compatibility with one another and their internal consistency (Rogers and Pilgrim, 2005). Existential psychologists such as Maslow (1968) developed the idea of 'self-actualization', which refers to each person fulfilling their human potential. But what if a person self-actualizes at the expense of the well-being of others? Similarly, a statistical norm can be used to define mental health but what of a society which contains unjust and destructive norms?

One recurrent difficulty with defining positive mental health is the same one that dogs the definition of mental illness or mental disorder: it is not easy to draw a firm line between normal and abnormal mental states. Differences in norms over time and place are the main undermining factor in such attempts. What is normal in one society may not be in another. Similarly, definitions of psychological normality and abnormality can vary over time in the same society. Is homosexuality a mental abnormality? Are hallucinations indicative of a spiritual gift or a mental illness? Posing these sorts of questions highlights the impermanent dividing line between mental health and mental abnormality;

- *'Mental health' as a prefix to describe one part of health services* Since the Second World War, the term 'mental health services' has now replaced that of 'psychiatric services' (though the latter is still sometimes used). Prior to the Second World War there were hospitals, clinics and asylums. These were either under parochial control, with a 'voluntary' or charitable history, or they served a specialist regional or national function. At that time though, they were not called 'services'. As Webster (1988) notes, prior to the NHS in Britain there was an admixture of charitable hospitals and medical relief offered to those in the workhouse system. This is why many of the older general hospitals were adapted poor house buildings. However, a major exception to this mixed picture was the network of dedicated mental illness and mental handicap hospitals which, since the Victorian period, had been funded and run by the State (Scull, 1979). The notion of a 'health service', post-1948 when the NHS was founded, reflects a shift towards a coherent system of organization and a notion of a publicly available resource (at the 'service' of the general population). Currently in Britain, specialist mental health services are either run by Primary Care Trusts or often (in the case of England) by specialist mental health/learning disability Trusts. In addition, there are privately run mental health facilities. These vary from small nursing homes to large hospitals which receive NHS patients who cannot be accommodated by local NHS mental health services. With devolution in the UK, specific policies about mental health service organization now vary from one country to another (Department of Health; 1998, 1999; Scottish Office, 1997; Welsh Assembly Government, 2002);
- *'Mental health' as a prefix to 'problems'* Just as the term 'mental

health services' has probably had a euphemistic value for those responsible for them (managers and politicians), the same is true of the term 'mental health problems'. By adding 'problems', to invert a notion of 'mental health', a less damning and stigmatizing state can be connoted. The professional discourse of diagnosis ('schizophrenia', 'bi-polar disorder' and so on) is stigmatizing. Indeed, sometimes psychiatrists simply do not communicate diagnoses such as these to their patients because of their negative connotations. In this context, the term 'mental health problems' may be less offensive to many parties. However, this might simply be a diversionary euphemism and it may not be persuasive as a tactic to avoid stigma for those with the label.

The terms 'mental health services' and 'mental health problems' may have been encouraged for additional reasons to those noted above. During the nineteenth century, all patients were certified under lunacy laws. That is, the State only made provisions for the control of madness. The fledgling profession of psychiatry (this term was first used in Britain in 1858) was singularly preoccupied with segregating and managing lunatics (Scull, 1979). With the emergence of the First World War, soldiers began to break down with 'shellshock' (now called 'post-traumatic stress disorder') (Stone, 1985). From this point on, psychiatry extended its jurisdiction from madness to versions of nervousness provoked by stress or trauma. Later, in the twentieth century, more abnormal mental states came within its jurisdiction, such as those due to alcohol and drug abuse and personality problems.

Today, 'mental health services' may be offered to, or be imposed upon, people with this wide range of problems, although madness or 'severe mental illness' still captures most of the attention of professionals. In this context, 'mental illness service' would be too narrow a description of the range of patients under psychiatric jurisdiction. The more accurate description, of 'mental disorder services', would be more inclusive. However, this term has not emerged in the English-speaking world. Also, the term 'psychiatric service' does not accurately reflect the multi-disciplinary nature of contemporary mental health work. So, for now, the term 'mental health service' serves as a compromise description. It avoids some inaccuracies but in some respects it is mystifying.

Another aspect of the term 'mental health problems' is that some people, critical of psychiatric terminology, object on scientific or logical grounds to notions like 'mental illness' or 'mental disorder'. An acceptable alternative for these critics is 'mental health problems', though another currently favoured alternative is 'mental distress'.

Thus, the use of the term 'mental health problems' side-steps the potential offence created by psychiatric diagnoses, given that the latter do not have scientific legitimacy for everyone.

See also: *fear; madness; psychiatric diagnosis; personality disorders and mental health promotion*

REFERENCES

Department of Health (1998) *Modernising Mental Health Services*. London: Department of Health.

Department of Health (1999) *A National Service Framework for Mental Health*. London: Department of Health.

Jahoda, M. (1958) *Current Concepts of Positive Mental Health*. New York: Basic Books.

Kubie, S. (1954) 'The fundamental nature of the distinction between normality and neurosis', *Psychoanalytical Quarterly*, 23: 167–204.

Maslow, A.H. (1968) *Toward a Psychology of Being*. Princeton, NJ: Princeton University Press.

Rogers, A. and Pilgrim, D. (2005) *A Sociology of Mental Health and Illness (Third Edition)*. Maidenhead: Open University Press.

Scottish Office (1997) *A Framework for Mental Health Services in Scotland*. Appendix to NHS MEL (1997) SODD Circular 30/97.

Scull, A. (1979) *Museums of Madness*. Harmondsworth: Penguin.

Stone, M. (1985) 'Shellshock and the psychologists', in W.E. Bynum, R. Porter and M. Shepherd (eds), *The Anatomy of Madness Vol 2*. London: Tavistock.

Webster, C. (1988) *The Health Services Since the War*. London: HMSO Books.

Welsh Assembly Government (2002) *Adult Mental Health Services: a National Service Framework for Wales*. Cardiff: Welsh Assembly Government.

World Health Organization (1951) *Technical Report Series (number 31)*. Geneva: WHO.

Psychiatric Diagnosis

***Definition:* The application of a medical label to a psychological abnormality.**

Key points: *• The history of psychiatric diagnosis is summarized • Criticisms of psychiatric diagnosis are rehearsed.*

During the nineteenth century, formal systems of diagnosis began to emerge in a variety of countries, as psychiatry developed as a specialism within medicine (Stone, 1997). Given that the new profession's main preoccupation was the management of lunacy, it focused on the codification of madness as a medical condition. For this reason, modern psychiatric classification is usually traced to Emil Kraepelin and his work on dementia praecox (soon re-labelled 'schizophrenia' by Eugen Bleuler) (see Bentall, 2003).

There had been many 'alienists' and 'mad-doctors' (terms used for medical specialists of the unbalanced mind) prior to Kraepelin, who had deliberated on diagnoses and their classifications, but most psychiatric textbooks now emphasize his seminal role. Currently there are two main medically accepted systems of psychiatric classification: the World Health Organization's (1992) *International Classification of Diseases (ICD)*; and the American Psychiatric Association's (1994) *Diagnostic and Statistical Manual of Mental Disorders (DSM)*. Both of these are reliant and build upon Kraepelin's work and his successor in German psychiatry, Kurt Schneider.

Kraepelin's first major medical description of 'dementia praecox' suggested an early deteriorating condition of the brain, which led to and maintained a state of madness from early adulthood onwards. Kraepelin began an important trend not only in medically codifying and classifying madness but in assuming a neurological basis for the condition. He enlisted the help of Alois Alzheimer, a neurologist, who had already found changes in the post-mortem brain tissue of some of those dementing in old age. It is still the case today that most psychiatrists consider that schizophrenia has genetically programmed neurological or bio-chemical bases. However, they are less pessimistic than Kraepelin and do not assume it to be an inevitably deteriorating chronic condition.

Scull (1979) has pointed out that the beginnings of medical authority over madness required a twin track professional strategy. The first was to wrest control of the lunatic asylums from lay administrators and establish a system of medical superintendents. The second was to install a form of classification, which asserted unambiguously that madness was a *bio-medical* condition. Scull quotes an editorial from the *Journal of Mental Science* (now the *British Journal of Psychiatry*) in 1858 which captures these points: 'madness is purely a condition of the brain. The physician is the guardian of the lunatic and must ever remain so'.

Today, assumptions about the biological origins of serious mental illness remain in a dominant position in psychiatry. However, its classification system eventually began to include conditions in which the primary role of biology was more ambiguous or even unlikely. For example, psychiatrists working with or as psychoanalysts developed a theory of neurosis which emphasized inter-personal and intra-psychic conflicts to account for mental abnormality. Also, behaviourist psychology began to provide its own environmentalist explanations for neurotic behaviour.

These psychological rather than biological accounts also led to a remaining and unresolved problem for psychiatry: the question of aetiology. The latter refers to the causes or origins of a pathological condition defined during a diagnosis. There are still strong disagreements between biological advocates and environmentalists. The biological, and still dominant, position is handicapped by its limited evidence base. For example, the bulk of diagnosed mental illnesses are still described as 'functional'. That is, they are based upon symptoms of speech and action not on bodily diagnostic signs. Because of these controversies, *DSM* at present makes no claim about aetiology and emphasizes, instead, behavioural descriptions of abnormal psychological conditions.

This limited descriptive emphasis can be criticized for its circularity. Symptoms are used to define a disorder but they are also accounted for by the presence of the disorder, using the following logic:

Q: how do you know this patient has schizophrenia?
A: because she lacks insight into her strange beliefs and she experiences auditory hallucinations.
Q: why does she have strange beliefs and experience hallucinations?
A: because she suffers from schizophrenia.

This circular logic is not a confident basis for making any diagnosis.

Since the days of Kraepelin, with his emphasis on madness (or psychosis), *DSM* and *ICD* have incorporated more and more diagnoses, which cover a range of phenomena, including forms of neurosis, personality problems, substance misuse and other forms of addictive behaviour. Of all those with these diagnoses, psychotic patients are defined by their lack of intelligibility to others and their lack of insight. By contrast, neurotic patients are aware that they have a problem (indeed it often becomes a preoccupation to them).

However, neat dividing lines, based upon intelligibility or insight, do not conveniently exist. A psychotic patient with a circumscribed delusion may act, for the most part, in a way that appears normal to others. A very obsessional neurotic patient may be deemed by others to lack insight into their condition and act in a visibly odd, rigid and ritualistic way. A patient with a diagnosis of anti-social personality disorder may act so outrageously that others may not understand it (calling it 'sick' or 'beyond belief' and so suggesting a criterion for psychosis). Thus, insight and intelligibility largely mark off psychosis from other forms of described mental disorder, but not unambiguously.

By the late twentieth century, Fish (1967) provided a basic psychiatric classification which still resonates in highly elaborated forms in more recent versions of *ICD* and *DSM*:

1 *Abnormal variations in mental life*
- abnormal intellectual endowments ('learning disability');
- abnormal personalities ('personality disorders');
- abnormal personality developments (e.g. the emergence of pathological jealousy);
- abnormal reactions to experience (e.g. 'post-traumatic stress disorder', neurotic distress, paranoid reactions).

2 *Mental illnesses*
- the functional psychoses (such as schizophrenia and bi-polar disorder);
- organic states (such as toxic reactions, drug-induced psychosis and some forms of senile dementia).

Under *DSM*, many versions of all of the above phenomena are subsumed under the single over-arching heading of 'mental disorder'. The latter includes a group missing from the list Fish (1967) constructed – people with addictive problems. As an indication of the uncertain state of psychiatric classification, while most psychiatrists today still would agree on the separation of organic from functional conditions, many would describe 'abnormal reactions to experience' as 'minor' or 'mild' mental illnesses.

A further complication about classification is that we cannot assume that symptom descriptions in the past match those used today. For example, Boyle (1991) studied the descriptions of symptoms used when diagnosing the patients of Kraepelin and Bleuler and found that they did not reflect the current symptom checklist to diagnose schizophrenia. This type of historical analysis casts doubt on whether modern psychiatry can offer a credible and stable classificatory system. So too do forms of analysis which focus on the reliability and validity of diagnosis.

Not only does the same patient often get diagnosed differently over time (indicating poor reliability of diagnosis) but patients with different diagnoses may have symptoms in common (poor conceptual validity). Validity problems are also seen within specific diagnoses. For example, schizophrenia is a disjunctive concept (Bannister, 1968) because two patients with the diagnosis may have no symptoms in common. Reliability can be improved by psychiatrists being trained carefully in the use of common symptom checklists (for example using *DSM*). However, *reliability* (consistency between diagnosticians and over time in the same patient) is not the same as *validity* (whether a diagnosis has objective evidence to confirm it and whether it is conceptually separate from other diagnostic categories). A third form of validity is predictive validity (a diagnosis should predict outcome of illness). Again this is highly imperfect in psychiatry, because human behaviour (of any sort) is difficult to predict accurately.

While a valid diagnosis has to have good reliability, it is possible to consistently use a label which is still not valid (Bentall, et al., 1988). These doubts about the validity and reliability of psychiatric diagnoses have led some to argue that mental disorder is very difficult to measure and that the dividing line between the normal and abnormal is fuzzy (Wakefield, 1999). As a consequence, estimating the incidence and prevalence of mental health problems becomes a precarious science.

A specific problem is pointed up by cross-cultural critics, who argue that judgements about what is normal or abnormal *ipso facto* reflect norms. If psychiatric diagnosis is about codifying non-conformity (rule breaking and role failure) in a particular culture, and cultures vary in their expectations of normal conduct, how can a stable and universal system of diagnosis be achieved? And when it is attempted (like in *DSM* and *ICD*) does this make it automatically insensitive to *particular* cultures in time and place?

Responses to these difficulties about the rationale for or the possibility of a stable universally valid system of psychiatric classification have varied:

- Defenders simply argue for a greater refinement of systems like *DSM* and *ICD* and their consistent use in medicine;
- Some critics argue for the wholesale rejection of psychiatric diagnostic categories in favour of individual formulations about presenting psychological difficulties. This criticism mainly comes from psychologists (e.g. Bruch and Bond, 1998);
- Some defenders point out that *DSM* has moved beyond simple categorization (the logic of a disorder being present or absent) and has included a *dimensional* view. This tension between a categorical view (e.g. a patient suffers from phobic anxiety) and a dimensional view (e.g. we are all, to some degree, phobic about something) fuels an ongoing debate about diagnosis within psychiatry (Kendell and Zealley, 1993);

- Some critics argue for the selective rejection of some types of people with difficulties from psychiatric jurisdiction. For example, some psychiatrists argue that only mental illness (psychotic and neurotic patterns of conduct) should fall within their remit. Those with acute transient distress, serious personality problems and substance misuse are not embraced and so are not really deemed to be worthy of formal psychiatric diagnosis. Other psychiatrists disagree and champion the treatment of these groups and so specialize in their diagnosis;
- Some psychiatrists accept the principle of diagnosis but emphasize cross-cultural sensitivity.

A final point to make about psychiatric diagnosis is that it is a product of psychiatry (as its name indicates). While madness, sadness and fear have always existed, as part of the human condition, 'mental illness', or 'mental disorder' only exist as by-products of psychiatric activity.

See also: *the 'myth of mental illness'; madness; sadness; fear; psychiatric epidemiology; substance misuse; personality disorders.*

REFERENCES

American Psychiatric Association (1994) *Diagnostic and Statistical Manual of Mental Disorders (Fourth Edition)*. Washington: APA.

Bannister, D. (1968) 'Logical requirements for research into schizophrenia', *British Journal of Psychiatry*, 114: 181–8.

Bentall, R.P. (2003) *Madness Explained*. London: Penguin.

Bentall, R.P., Pilgrim, D. and Jackson, H. (1988) 'Abandoning the concept of schizophrenia: some implications of validity arguments for psychological research into psychotic phenomena', *British Journal of Clinical Psychology*, 27: 303–24.

Boyle, M. (1991) *Schizophrenia: a Scientific Delusion?* London: Routledge.

Bruch, M. and Bond, F.W. (eds) (1998) *Beyond Diagnosis: Case Formulation Approaches in CBT*. London: Wiley.

Fish, F. (1967) *Clinical Psychopathology: Signs and Symptoms in Psychiatry*. Bristol: John Wright and Sons.

Kendell, R.E. and Zealley, A.K. (1993) *Companion to Psychiatric Studies*. Edinburgh: Churchill Livingstone.

Scull, A. (1979) *Museums of Madness*. Harmondsworth: Penguin.

Stone, M.H. (1997) *Healing the Mind: a History of Psychiatry from Antiquity to the Present*. New York: Norton.

Wakefield, J.C. (1999) 'The measurement of mental disorder', in A.V. Horwitz and T.L. Scheid (eds), *A Handbook for the Study of Mental Health*. Cambridge: Cambridge University Press.

World Health Organization (1992) *The ICD-10 Classification of Mental and Behavioural Disorders*. Geneva: WHO.

Psychiatric Epidemiology

Definition: The study of the incidence and prevalence of mental disorder in time and space.

Key points: • *Psychiatric epidemiology is described* • *Its weakness compared to traditional medical epidemiology is discussed.*

In medicine, incidence refers to the number of new or first cases diagnosed. Prevalence refers to the total number of cases present in a population at a point in time or for a specified period of time. Epidemiology is the study of incidence and prevalence of diseases in space and time. Estimates of both prevalence and incidence of mental disorders are not easy for the following reasons:

1 Some critics argue that it is inappropriate to count cases, other than those with true organic conditions, which are associated with psychological abnormality (Szasz, 1961);
2 Critics who, in principle, accept the legitimacy of functional psychiatric diagnoses concede that particular diagnostic categories suffer from validity problems (Wakefield, 1999). These validity problems undermine our confidence in what is being counted;
3 In the absence of a consensus about the aetiology of most functional mental illnesses, the best that can be achieved by psychiatric epidemiology is to map the number of cases. It cannot achieve a causal map. This can be contrasted with the stronger tradition of medical epidemiology, in which causes not just cases are mapped. An example would be mapping the geographical spread of the incidence or prevalence of an infectious disease, such as tuberculosis. Psychiatric epidemiology is thus *descriptive* at best. It may be able to describe correlations between social variables (say social class, gender and race) and mental disorder.

However, correlations may not imply causality and even it they do, as in the case of social class position, the direction of causality may be disputed.

The problems of valid and reliable case identification in psychiatric epidemiology are summed up well here:

> Epidemiology is a branch of medicine and thus the assumptions of the medical model of disease are implicit. The most important assumption is that the disease under study actually exists. In psychiatry this assumption is assuredly more tenuous than in other areas of medicine, because psychiatric diseases tend to be defined by a failure to locate a physical cause, and a validation of a given category of disease is therefore more subtle and complex. (Eaton, 1986)

With this type of caution in mind, what estimates are given by the psychiatric literature? The criticisms are confirmed by quite large variations in published estimates. For example, a review of eight US studies of prevalence estimates of personality disorder (all types) found a range of 6–15% in the general population and up to 50% in clinical psychiatric populations (de Girolamo and Dotto, 2000). Some studies find that borderline and histrionic personality disorders are more common in women but others find no sex differences. Much of this variation seems to reflect differences in diagnostic measures.

Variable estimates are also found in anxiety-based disorders. For example, community samples suggest a one-year prevalence of 7% for women and 9% for men of social phobia but clinical samples suggest no sex differences (Kessler et al., 1994). In the latter study, much larger sex differences were found in community samples for panic disorder (1.3% for men and 3.2% for women). Although most studies show a lifetime prevalence of obsessive-compulsive disorder of around 2%, estimates vary in different parts of the world from 1–3% (Weissman et al., 1994). Of course variations may represent real differences rather than artefacts of measurement. The problem is that it is not easy to resolve which of these two possibilities is most likely, given the concerns about the validity of particular diagnoses noted earlier from the likes of Szasz, Eaton and Wakefield.

If the validity of diagnoses of schizophrenia and bi-polar disorder is accepted then variations are still found. The lifetime risk of bi-polar disorder ranges from 0.3% to 1.5% with no discernible sex differences (Kessler et al., 1997). When those with a diagnosis of schizophrenia have been studied, the annual incidence lies between 0.017 and 0.54%, with a one-year prevalence ranging from 0.14% to 0.46% (Jablensky, 2000). Within these figures large racial differences appear (for example with a higher incidence in young Afro-Caribbean men in Britain).

A final question about psychiatric epidemiology relates to its social administrative role. Given its descriptive character, it has been largely used by psychiatrists and some policy makers to define *need for services*. That is, by estimating the prevalence of disorders separately and together mental health service provision can be planned. The apparently benign role of service planning is not without its critics, given that mental health services are linked to coercion, stigma and social exclusion. This can lead to people with mental health problems evading services rather than demanding them.

See also: *psychiatric diagnosis; mental health; coercion; stigma; social exclusion; race; the 'myth of mental illness'.*

REFERENCES

de Girolamo, G. and Dotto, P. (2000) 'Epidemiology of personality disorders', in M.G. Gelder, J.J. Lopez-Ibor and N.C. Andreasen (eds), *The New Oxford Textbook of Psychiatry.* Oxford: Oxford University Press.

Eaton, W. (1986) *The Sociology of Mental Disorders*. New York: Praeger.

Jablensky, A. (2000) 'Epidemiology of schizophrenia', in M.G. Gelder, J.J. Lopez-Ibor and N.C. Andreasen (eds), *The New Oxford Textbook of Psychiatry*. Oxford: Oxford University Press.

Kessler, R.C., McGonagle, K.A. and Zhao, S. (1994) 'Lifetime and 12-month prevalence of DSM-II-R psychiatric disorders in the United States: results from the National Comorbidity Survey', *Archives of General Psychiatry*, 51: 8–20.

Kessler, R.C., Rubinow, D.R. and Holmes, C. (1997) 'The epidemiology of DSM-III-R bipolar I disorder in a general population survey', *Psychological Medicine*, 27: 1079–89.

Szasz, T.S. (1961) *The Myth of Mental Illness: Foundations of Theory of Personal Conduct*. New York: Harper & Row.

Wakefield, J.C. (1999) 'The measurement of mental disorder', in A.V. Horwitz and T.L. Scheid (eds), *A Handbook for the Study of Mental Health.* Cambridge: Cambridge University Press.

Weissman, M.M., Bland, R.C. and Canino, G.J. (1994) 'The gross national epidemiology of obsessive-compulsive disorders', *Journal of Clinical Psychiatry*, 55: 5–11.

Functional and Organic Mental Illnesses

Definition: Functional mental illnesses are defined by abnormalities of speech and action (symptoms), whereas organic mental illnesses are defined by observable or measurable bodily abnormalities (signs) in addition to symptoms.

Key points: • *The traditional distinction between organic and functional psychiatric diagnoses is explained* • *Examples of organic and functional conditions are provided.*

The division between functional and organic mental illnesses by psychiatrists is now well established. However, one wing of the profession (biological psychiatry or neuropsychiatry) tends to assume that *all* mental illnesses are caused by some form of biological malfunction. This can be thought of as a form of 'hoped-for-reductionism'. It is best expressed by one of its main contemporary champions, Samuel Guze. Here he makes this point clearly:

> . . . what is called psychopathology *is* the manifestation of disordered processes in various brain systems that mediate psychological functioning . . . By taking into consideration genetic codes and epigenetic development, guided and shaped by broad ranging environmental influences, only some of which are now recognised and understood, biology *clearly offers* the *only* comprehensive basis for psychiatry just as it does for the rest of medicine. (Guze, 1989: 317–18, emphasis added)

The certainty expressed by Guze is not shared by all psychiatrists though. Many have an open mind about aetiology in psychiatric diagnosis. Consequently, they retain an emphasis upon defining one group of illnesses as 'functional' and another as 'organic'. In the latter, bodily signs indicate either a temporary chemical disturbance (for example a psychotic reaction to amphetamine use) or structural changes in the brain (for example in Alzheimer's disease). By contrast, bodily signs are either markedly absent or a matter of conjecture and debate in the case of functional conditions.

Clinicians will also mention that they have a different sense about the 'organic' patient's symptoms. For example, while hallucinations are present in both drug-induced psychosis and in many with a diagnosis of schizophrenia, the former tends to have visual and the latter auditory hallucinations. Also cognitive deficits (delirium, restricted reasoning power, short-term memory loss and disorientation in time and space) are more pronounced in organic conditions and may even be the only symptoms present.

However, these distinctions are not hard and fast. For example, personality changes in a patient often indicate a neurological change. But some patients diagnosed with schizophrenia or post-traumatic stress disorder also show personality changes. Or extending an example already given, visual hallucinations and delirium are common in drug-induced states but can also be found in histrionic patients at times. A good example of the latter is 'prison psychosis', where a recently arrested criminal attempts to avoid responsibility for their crime by presenting with wild and delirious symptoms or with psychotic mutism (staring ahead and refusing to speak). Also, dementing patients may need to die before organic damage can definitely be identified *post-mortem*. While they are alive, it is still a range of functional problems (about their conduct indicating problems of memory and orientation) which drive the diagnosis. Thus, as with other debates about neat dividing lines in the field of mental health, the one dividing and defining organic and functional patients is also fuzzy.

DSM-IV (American Psychiatric Association, 1994) divided organic mental disorders into three main types:

1 *Delirium* resulting from medical illness (such as fever), drug use or drug withdrawal;
2 *Dementia* resulting from changes in the brain's tissue (due to loss or injury from a variety of causes, some known, some not);
3 *Amnestic disorders* where memory loss predominates and is caused by medical conditions or excessive or chronic substance misuse.

The functional mental illnesses described as 'major', 'serious' or 'severe' are those allotted to patients with diagnoses of schizophrenia or bi-polar disorder (sometimes still called 'manic-depressive' illness, psychosis or disorder). These represent modern medical codifications of madness. In the case of the diagnosis of schizophrenia, *DSM-IV* stipulates six criteria:

1 In the active phase there are two or more of the following: delusions, hallucinations, disorganized speech ('thought disorder'), disorganized behaviour or catatonia (mute rigidity) and negative symptoms (flat emotions and loss of motivation);
2 In the lead up to the diagnosis there should have been evidence of marked disturbance in one or more of the following areas of life: poor functioning at work or school, disturbed personal relationships or social withdrawal, poor self-care;
3 The above disturbance must have been present for at least six months (with at least one month of active symptoms);
4 Disturbances of mood should be excluded as an alternative diagnosis (see bi-polar disorder below);
5 Substance misuse or medical explanations for the symptoms must be excluded;
6 Those with a pre-existing developmental disorder (such as autism) should be excluded.

This is the official starting checklist, but psychiatrists then vary in their sympathy for a whole range of sub-divisions of the condition. Some include paranoid psychosis as a part of schizophrenia; others see it as a separate condition (Gelder et al., 2001).

Turning to the diagnosis of mood disorders, these may be transient and may not be considered to reach psychotic proportions by others. In those with a diagnosis of bi-polar disorder, patients are deemed to oscillate between extremes of depression and mania. In the former state, the patient is paralysed by sadness and self-deprecation. They may enter a slow stupor and refuse to eat or drink. They may try to commit suicide or express the intense desire to do so. In the manic phase the patient becomes elated and expansive in their thoughts and ambitions. Their thoughts, expressed in speech, are fast and furious and others have difficulty tracking their meaning ('flight of ideas'). Also, they may express grandiose delusions about their powers and abilities.

Other functional disorders are deemed to be mainly a result of the patient dealing with anxiety in their life (e.g. phobic-anxiety, histrionic reactions and generalized anxiety disorder). These are described further in the section on fear. Whether anxiety-based disorders should be called 'mild to moderate functional mental illnesses', or 'abnormal variations' in mental life, remains a moot point.

See also: *psychiatric diagnosis; fear; causes and constructs; sadness.*

REFERENCES

American Psychiatric Association (1994) *Diagnostic and Statistical Manual of Mental Disorders (Fourth Edition)*. Washington: APA.

Gelder, M., Mayou, R. and Cowen, P. (2001) *Shorter Oxford Textbook of Psychiatry*. Oxford: Oxford University Press.

Guze, S. (1989) 'Biological psychiatry: is there any other kind?', *Psychological Medicine*, 19: 315–23.

Madness

***Definition:* Madness is sustained unintelligible conduct. The mad person inhabits an idiosyncratic world, which does not make immediate sense to others.**

Key points: • *The relationship between lay and professional descriptions of madness is discussed* • *The merits of non-medical ways of framing madness are examined.*

Madness has also officially been called 'lunacy' and 'insanity'. The latter is still used in our legal system but the former is now defunct. Since the nineteenth century, mental health professionals have also used 'mania', 'melancholia', 'psychosis', 'schizophrenia', 'manic-depression', 'schizo-affective disorder' and 'bi-polar disorder'. This emphasizes the shifting ways in which the English language frames madness in the official world of politicians and clinicians.

Such is the fear or amusement that madness creates in the general population that we have quite a rich lexicon to describe it. Terms used in the English vernacular about madness have included 'crazy', 'crackers', 'deranged', 'bonkers', 'batty', 'bananas', 'psycho', 'potty', 'do-lally', 'away with the fairies', 'on another planet', 'spacey', 'loony', 'loopy', 'touched', 'wacky' or just 'mental'. The latter connotation has meant that those with learning disabilities (what was called '*mental* handicap') have also been stereotyped as being mad. This reflects an ancient conflation of madness and foolishness. Since the English language readily draws on foreign sources at times, we also have: to go 'loco' (from Spain); or 'berserk' (from Scandinavia); or to run 'amok' (from South Asia).

Many of the disparaging lay terms used above imply alienation (with the mad being under extra-planetary influence or being strangers to themselves or the rest of humanity). For many years, experts on madness were called 'alienists'. In the madhouses of the seventeenth and eighteenth century, the mad were seen as not really human and so they could be visited and viewed with horror or amusement by normal citizens, without any sense of guilt or remorse.

Although 'severe mental illness', 'psychosis', 'schizophrenia' or 'bi-polar disorder' only began to exist with the emergence of the psychiatric profession, as its preferred codifications of madness, the latter has always existed. This point is made to emphasize that madness is not simply a slippery semantic construction. There does seem to have been a real and consistent pattern of description across the centuries. Since antiquity records of various societies indicate that those who transgress social expectations, in ways which others cannot fathom, provoke some clear description of difference.

Two stereotypical and enduring descriptions of madness since ancient times have included violence and aimless wandering. Other features include mad people talking to themselves (outside of an intelligible religious ritual or context of prayer) and expressing grandiose or ridiculous views, which the challenges of others do not modify. Madness has also invited emotional descriptions of being wild and exuberant or flat and dejected, in contexts in which these forms of expression were unexpected. In accord with the violent stereotype of madness, the word 'mad' also means furiously angry.

Before madness became medicalized in the nineteenth century, it was described and explained within moral and supernatural frameworks. The early asylum system was run by religious lay people who saw madness as evidence of demonic possession or influence, leading to corruption of the soul and the ensuing animalistic deterioration of the personality. For this reason, 'moral treatment' was the first systematic attempt to bring the insane back into the fold of normal society.

Although scientific medicine is critical of this outmoded view, it did locate madness in a moral context. To re-frame it as mental illness (the current Western rational medical view) de-contextualizes mad conduct and attributes it to essential pathology within the individual. More strongly than this, it attributes it to some yet to be discovered disorder of the brain and pre-empts the possibility that madness might actually be meaningful, even if not in an immediate sense. By contrast, the older view meant that the mad person's actions were being evaluated within a moral and religious framework. Thus the latter, not just the person, was open to interpretation or interrogation.

The clinical gaze of the psychiatric profession encourages us only to look at individuals as manifestations of mental illness and not the profession that claims expertise about them or those parties in society in whose interests it works. It is as if simply to describe symptoms of mental illness as pathology (and so meaningless communication) is all that is required in order to describe madness. This closes down rather than opens up an exploration of the mystery of madness and its regular negotiation by those who remain sane by common consent.

The religious framing of madness as negative or demonic has been far from unambiguous. Religious exuberance ('religiosity') has been seen as divine or inspired at times rather than devilish. Examples of this today can be found in some forms of ultra-orthodox Judaism. Similarly, religious madness was associated with positive protestant revivalism in Northern Ireland during the mid-nineteenth century. The capacity to 'talk in tongues' has been framed as divine, not demonic, intervention in Pentecostal Christian sects. The Greek philosopher Socrates pointed out the equal value of sanity and madness, because good forms of the latter were supplied by the gods. He emphasized the positive aspects of mad rapture: prophesying (a 'manic art'); mystical initiations and rituals; poetic inspiration; and the 'madness' of mutual lovers. All of these points resonate in religious belief systems today. They are also a corrective to the negative view that madness is merely a comical, frightening or pitiful state.

In some cultures, some of the symptoms of madness (particularly the experience of hallucinations and thought insertion, where an idea comes to mind from an outside source) have been seen as a supernatural gift shown by shamans and religious leaders, rather than a defect or malady. Saints, prophets and pious hermits have also shown clear signs of madness, with their visions and claims of clairvoyance. Their claims of peculiar religious insights and their withdrawal from normal society would now readily invite a diagnosis of severe mental illness.

Madness is defined by the attributions of others and the transgression of the fundamental rule in adult society of being able to render one's behaviour intelligible to others when required. This 'intelligibility rule' is a characteristic of societies not individuals. Consequently, madness is a social judgement not a medical-scientific fact. Moreover, not only are exceptions tolerated to the intelligibility rule, to various degrees in various societies but conformity to the rules of reason or rationality does not always produce healthy outcomes.

It is true that mad people are unintelligible to others and so lack credibility as citizens. However, it is also true that sane people may act reasonably and intelligibly but be highly destructive. The threats of warfare and ecological degradation to humanity as a whole, the pursuit of genocide and the building of concentration camps have been the collective outcome of sane people acting in a reasonable and intelligible way, according to the norms of their parent society.

In other words, the disvalue that is placed on the irrationality of individuals is only one way of attributing pathology. Descriptions of pathology ultimately are value judgements and health can be defined perversely as conformity to an unhealthy society. Rationality, transparency and efficiency (the ideal features of normal people in modern industrialized societies) taken to their ultimate conclusions can also be pathological. For this reason, many of those hostile to a naïve mental illness view of madness have argued for concerted efforts to create productive conversations between normality and madness, with the assumption that advantages might accrue in both directions. Relevant examples here were of the works of Ronald Laing and Michel Foucault, who noted that in modern societies, the dialogue between reason and unreason has broken down. According to Laing's colleague, David Cooper, this broken dialogue now means that the opposite of madness is not sanity but normality.

See also: *the 'myth of mental illness'; psychiatric diagnosis; creativity; causes and constructs; 'anti-psychiatry'.*

FURTHER READING

Cooper, D. (1968) *Psychiatry and Anti-Psychiatry*. London: Tavistock.
Coulter, J. (1973) *Approaches to Insanity*. New York: Wiley.
Donay, J.G. (1985) 'Medicine and religion: on the physical and mental disorders that accompanied the Ulster Revival of 1859', in W.F. Bynum, R. Porter and M. Shepherd (eds), *The Anatomy of Madness Vol III*. London: Tavistock.
Foucault, M. (1965) *Madness and Civilisation*. New York: Random House.
Fromm, E. (1955) *The Sane Society*. New York: Holt, Reinhart and Winston.
Laing, R.D. (1967) *The Politics of Experience and the Bird of Paradise*. Harmondsworth: Penguin.
Porter, R. (1989) *A Social History of Madness*. London: Routledge.
Rosen, G. (1968) *Madness in Society*. New York: Harper.
Screech, M.A. (1985) 'Good madness in Christendom', in W.F. Bynum, R. Porter and M. Shepherd (eds), *The Anatomy of Madness (Volume I)*. London: Tavistock.
Scull, A.(1979) *Museums of Madness*. London: Allen Lane.
Wing, J. (1978) *Reasoning About Madness*. Oxford: Oxford University Press.

Sadness

Definition: Sadness is a state of mournful sorrow.

Key points: *• Sadness and depression are discussed • The problem of cultural relativism in describing emotional states is outlined • Criticisms of the psychiatric diagnosis of depression are summarized.*

In the *Oxford English Dictionary*, one of the meanings of 'depression' is described as: '(Psych.) state of morbidly excessive melancholy, mood of hopelessness and feelings of inadequacy often with physical symptoms'. Here, deliberately, we start not with depression but with sadness. Because the word 'depression' has now entered the vernacular, even though the dictionary indicates it to be a technical term from psychiatry, sadness will be explored first. A discussion of the meaning of depression will then follow.

Feelings of any sort are experienced and then possibly expressed with words. Words themselves shape what it is legitimate to feel and not feel. As words reflect thoughts, once they are learned after infancy they typically merge with feelings in a person's experience. The words available to describe feelings vary from culture to culture. In English there are around 2000 words to describe feelings, though only around 200 are in common use (Wallace and Carson, 1973). By contrast, the Ifalukians of Micronesia have only 58 words to describe transient internal states (Lutz, 1980) and the Chewong of Malaysia have only seven words which translate into English words about emotions (Howell, 1981). Russell (1991) found than in some African languages a single word is used to mean both 'anger' and 'sadness' in English translation.

When asked to look at emotional expressions in human faces, North American and Japanese subjects agree on 'sadness' and 'surprise' but not on 'anger' or 'fear'. These differences should lead us to be cautious about assuming that technical terms in Anglo-American psychiatry, related to mood states, have universal applicability. Because of the richness of the English language, we may also assume that other languages are more restricted in their emotional descriptions, but this is not always the case. For example, we do not have good words in English to capture the German notions of 'angst' or 'schadenfreude' – hence our tendency to leave them untranslated, while having a general sense of their meaning.

With this caution about cultural differences in mind, Russell (1991) in his cross-cultural comparisons concluded that there were indeed some universal emotional states. These can be roughly translated onto this emotional circumflex based on two dimensions using ordinary words of the English language, with equivalents in the majority of others:

Figure 1 *The emotional circumplex* (Russell, 1991)

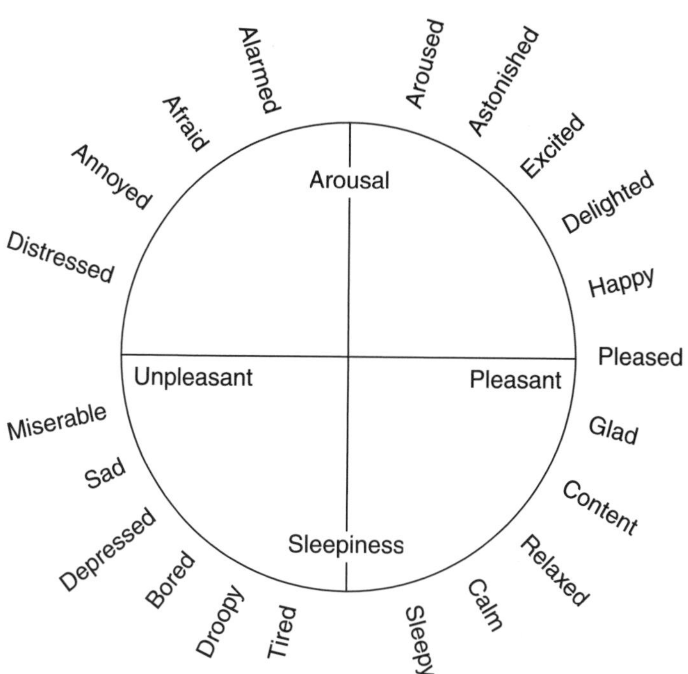

For our purposes here it should be noted that being sad seems to be a universal state. It is probably also fair to assume that the state is not peculiarly human. All higher mammals seem to show signs of sadness under conditions of loss or learned helplessness. (Seligman, 1975)

Because it is an unpleasant state, a related matter is whether distressing sadness should be suppressed or simply left to persist or disappear without intervention. Here again cultural differences come into play. Cultures vary in their expectations of how long and how profoundly we should mourn the loss of others. Buddhists argue that suffering (with sadness being one of its manifestations) is inherent to the human condition. Likewise, existentialists argue that we should stay with discomforting feelings (like sadness and anxiety) in order to confront their source and meaning in our lives. By technicalizing this form of suffering as an illness and invoking medical paternalism to remove it (for example by using 'anti-depressant' drugs), arguably we are party to a form of rationalistic arrogance and cultural imperialism.

Turning then to the term 'depression', its meaning is not consistent in Western psychiatry, nor is it preferred by psychiatrists universally. For example in China both psychiatrists and lay people use the notion of 'neurasthenia' in preference to 'depression'. The term 'neurasthenia' was used in English psychiatry in the nineteenth century to describe nervous fatigue but is now obsolete in the West (Kleinman, 1988). Anglo-American psychiatry currently agrees that depression is its 'common cold' – the diagnosis of greatest prevalence – but it still does not agree consistently on its meaning. Pilgrim and Bentall (1999) reviewed a variety of authoritative psychiatric texts and found the following:

- Some major texts do not even define depression (e.g. Beck et al., 1979; Golden and Janowsky, 1990). This may imply that the concept has self-evident validity for the authors and requires no formal description;
- Some texts argue that depression is primarily a disturbance of *mood* with all other features (cognitive symptoms like negativism and somatic ones like poor appetite) being secondary to this (e.g. Becker, 1977; Lewis, 1934);
- Other texts argue that it is primarily defined by *cognitive* features – a negative view of self, the world and the future (e.g. Beck et al., 1979);
- There is no agreement on whether depression is an illness, a syndrome, a mood or a symptom (cf. Davison and Neale, 1990; Montgomery, 1990);
- While *DSM-IV* (American Psychiatric Association, 1994) demands the presence of depressed mood plus four other symptoms for a diagnosis of major depression, some other North American authorities offer a wider range of symptoms but argue that none, *not even depressed mood*, is essential for the diagnosis (e.g. Willner, 1985);

- A final complication is that mild to moderate ('neurotic') depression is often co-present with anxiety, with some texts consequently arguing that a unified diagnosis of a 'general neurotic syndrome' should replace both (e.g. Goldberg and Huxley, 1992; Tyrer, 1990).

Thus, what starts as an apparently obvious consensus, that depression is the commonest of all mental disorders and that is understood well now by lay people, as well as mental health professionals, turns out to be problematic. We cannot assume that our Western view of depressive illness has universal applicability. Nor can we assume that psychiatrists have a strong agreement about what they mean by 'depression'. Claims that 'clinical depression' is categorically different from 'dysphoria', or 'everyday unhappiness', cannot be demonstrated readily. Despite the difficulties surrounding the conceptual validity of 'depression' (or maybe in part because of its woolly inclusiveness) epidemiologists now record it as being the fourth largest contributor to the global burden of disease – a role that is considered to be rising (Murray and Lopez, 1995).

None of the above critical discussion is to argue that people cannot be profoundly sad and that this experience is not life diminishing or even at times life threatening. However, it does query whether the use of the word 'depression', as a medical codification of 'sadness' or 'misery', offers us clarity or improves our understanding of a universally experienced and extremely common aspect of human suffering.

See also: *fear; madness; causes and constructs.*

REFERENCES

American Psychiatric Association (1994) *Diagnostic and Statistical Manual of Mental Disorders (Fourth Edition)*. Washington: APA.

Beck, A.T., Rush, A.J., Shaw, B.F. and Emery, G.(1979) *Cognitive Therapy of Depression*. New York: Guilford Press.

Becker, J. (1977) *Affective Disorders*. Morristown, NJ: General Learning Press.

Davison, G.C. and Neale, J.M. (1990) *Abnormal Psychology*. New York: Wiley.

Goldberg, D. and Huxley, P. (1992) *Common Mental Disorders: a Bio-social Model*. London: Routledge.

Golden, R.N. and Janowsky, D.S. (1990) 'Biological theories of depression', in B.B. Wolman and G. Stricker (eds), *Depressive Disorders*. New York: Wiley.

Howell, S. (1981) 'Rules not words', in P. Heelas and A. Lock (eds), *Indigenous Psychologies: the Anthropology of the Self*. San Diego, CA: Academic Press.

Kleinman, A. (1988) *Rethinking Psychiatry*. New York: Free Press.

Lewis, A. (1934) 'Melancholia: a clinical survey of depressive states', *Journal of Mental Science*, 80: 227–78.

Lutz, C. (1980) 'Emotion words and emotional development'. Unpublished PhD dissertation, University of Harvard, MA.
Montgomery, S. (1990) *Anxiety and Depression*. London: Livingstone.
Murray, C.J.L. and Lopez, A.D. (eds) (1995) *The Global Burden of Disease*. Cambridge, MA: Harvard University Press.
Pilgrim, D. and Bentall, R.P. (1999) 'The medicalisation of misery: a critical realist analysis of the concept of depression', *Journal of Mental Health*, 8 (3): 261–74.
Russell, J.A. (1991) 'A circumflex model of affect', *Journal of Personality and Social Psychology*, 45: 848–56.
Seligman, M.E.P. (1975) *Helplessness: on Depression, Development and Death*. San Francisco: Freeman.
Tyrer, P. (1990) 'The division of neurosis: a failed classification', *Journal of the Royal Society of Medicine*, 83: 614–16.
Wallace, A.F.C. and Carson, M.T. (1973) 'Sharing and diversity in emotional terminology', *Ethos*, 1: 1–29.
Willner, P. (1985) *Depression: a Psychobiological Synthesis*. New York: Wiley.

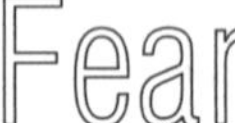

Fear

***Definition:* Fear is the behaviour and experience provoked in humans and other animals by real or perceived threats.**

Key points: *• Fear and anxiety are described • The psychiatric codification of anxiety based problems is discussed.*

Fear is a normal physiological and behavioural response to threat, evident in most animals. The term 'anxiety' is usually described as 'irrational fear', but the experience is still one of fear. Anxiety is manifested directly in humans in a range of symptoms. These include cognitive disturbances (such as poor concentration, irritability, a sense of impending doom or 'free floating anxiety'), autonomic arousal (such as sweating, dry mouth and palpitations), muscle tension, hyperventilation and sleep disturbances. The permutation of these various symptoms varies from one anxious person to another.

Traditionally, anxious and depressed patients are described as 'neurotic' personalities if their symptoms are chronic or as having 'neurotic reactions' if not. In the vernacular, neurotic reactions are often called 'nervous breakdowns'. Neurotic patients are distressed and conscious of, or even preoccupied with, their symptoms. In all other respects they are deemed to be rational and coherent and they are able to relate successfully to others. This traditionally differentiates the neuroses from the psychoses.

However, the boundary between neurosis and other states is not fixed. At times neurotic patients may be deemed to lack insight and they may become a-social in their behaviour. Also, when neurotic symptoms become chronic and resistant to treatment the patient may be re-classified as being 'personality disordered'. For example, those with chronic obsessive-compulsive symptoms who fail to respond to treatment may be re-classified as suffering from 'obsessive-compulsive personality disorder'. Similarly, the chronic social phobic might be thought of as suffering from an 'anxious avoidant personality disorder'.

Current psychiatric classification systems like *DSM* and *ICD* divide the broad field of anxiety neurosis into three groups, which subsume types:

- phobic anxiety disorders (agoraphobia, with or without panic disorder, social phobia and specific phobias);
- panic disorder (without agoraphobia);
- anxiety disorder (generalized; obsessive-compulsive (under *DSM* but *ICD* places it as a separate disorder), mixed with depression (*ICD* only)).

Sigmund Freud distinguished between objective anxiety (a function of external threat) and subjective anxiety, which was derived from internal conflicts. In the latter case he pointed in a general sense to the conflict between the instincts (sexual energy or libido, to which he later added the death instinct) and the socially required rationality and morality demanded of civilized adults.

The term 'anxiety' tends to be limited to humans but can be created experimentally in other mammals. The earliest demonstration of this was by Ivan Pavlov, who gave shocks to dogs unpredictably under conditions in which they could not escape. This began a behaviourist tradition of viewing anxiety as a conditioned fear response.

However anxiety is explained, in the field of mental health it is seen as the core common characteristic of neurotic presentations, if depression is excluded. Moreover, both the psychoanalytical and behaviourist traditions view anxiety as developmentally derived and pervasive. Freud considered that we were all, to some degree, neurotic. Psychoanalysis views us all as ill, with anxiety neurosis being the price we pay for living in a rule-bound civilized world. Similarly, behaviourists would argue that we are all frightened of something to some degree.

Eventually behaviourists conceded that anxiety and other emotions implicated thoughts, not just behaviour (reducing the gap between the objective emphasis in behaviourism and the subjective emphasis in psychoanalysis). This has led to a modification of the treatment of neurosis, within the behaviourist tradition. Previously, the emphasis was narrowly on the modification of fearful behaviour – an example of this was the gradual exposure of the person to the object evoking their fear ('systematic desensitization'). Now behavioural methods have been overtaken by cognitive-behavioural therapy, which works with inner life as well as external responses.

Existential therapists take a different view of anxiety. Rather than seeking to remove it as a form of distress (the behavioural view) or seeking a common understanding with the patient of its historical source (the psychoanalytical view), the existentialist would ask the patient to tolerate it, rather than remove or explain it. From this process the patient is offered an opportunity to discover meaning in the ambiguity of the anxious experience. Existentialists view anxiety, like Buddhists view suffering, as integral to the human condition rather than as an exceptional state (what Søren Kierkegaard called 'sickness unto death').

The sociological questions that arise from these general psychological statements relate to why some people experience this or that form of anxiety in a particular context. Take the example of agoraphobia – panic or strong insecurity when away from a patient's home base. In the wake of industrialization, this emerged in crowded urban areas with the new threats this brought, especially to women. The diagnosis is still given to twice as many women as men. Public spaces are more risky in complex urban areas than in quiet rural villages. All forms of anxiety symptoms increase in probability in the wake of social stress or specific trauma. As a consequence, the social antecedents of an anxious presentation are important to understand. For example, domestic violence and other violent crimes predict the development of panic disorder in victims.

The preference of the medical profession for drug treatments and the high prevalence of anxiety symptoms in the general population led to problems about their use. Drugs targeting anxiety are called anxiolytics and the largest group of these, the benzodiazepines, dominated the market between 1960 and the 1980s. These were very addictive and were ineffective at symptom reduction after a few weeks. This created an iatrogenic epidemic of addiction, with no long-term mental health gain for the patients receiving the drugs. Professionally led and self-help groups then had to be set up to help people to come off the drugs. Since then low dose anti-depressants have been used as an alternative, as well as drugs altering autonomic nervous system activity, such as beta-blockers.

The descriptions given under *DSM* and *ICD* above focus only on those diagnoses in which anxiety is directly experienced and overtly expressed by the patient. Apart from *ICD* separating obsessive-compulsive disorder (OCD), both systems deal with other indications of the role of anxiety, even if they are formally described outside of the domain of the anxiety disorders. Freud's original interest in hysteria (now described as 'histrionic' reaction or personality and 'somatization' and 'hypochondriasis'), as a pure form of neurosis, raises an important question: is anxiety at the heart of *all* forms of mental abnormality?

Certainly psychological theories of psychosis are now emphasizing the role of underlying trauma and anxiety (for example see Richard Bentall's *Madness Explained*). Some psychoanalysts, like Ronald Fairbairn and Harry Guntrip suggested that all psychopathology is about the anxious struggle to preserve the ego. Others, like John Bowlby, also focused on the role of actual or anticipated loss or separation being a recurrent source of anxiety as well as depression in human beings. While these views about the role of anxiety in depressive, psychotic and schizoid phenomena remain contentious, in the cases of OCD, histrionic behaviour and hypochondriasis the patient is involved in barely veiled attempts to deal with the pain of anxiety.

The professional jurisdiction over anxiety disorders has shifted over the years. During the late nineteenth century, as the psychiatric profession established itself, it took very little interest in neurosis and was preoccupied with lunacy. The shellshock problem of the First World War altered this focus. However, the treatment of neurosis remained split off in the private consulting worlds of the psychotherapist, military treatment centres or in metropolitan specialist facilities like the Tavistock Clinic.

After the Second World War, mental health professionals in the NHS began to take more and more interest in anxiety problems, with clinical psychologists, nurse therapists and some psychiatrists championing their treatment using psychological therapies. The treatment of anxiety problems is now common in mental health services but most patients presenting with these difficulties are not referred to specialist services, with the demand for the latter well outstripping supply. As a result, experiments with community-based self-help and computerized systems of treatment are becoming more common, particularly as confidence in drug treatments has been undermined by the benzodiazepine-dependence problem noted earlier.

See also: *psychiatric diagnosis; sadness; causes and constructs; personality disorders.*

FURTHER READING

Bentall, R.P. (2003) *Madness Explained*. London: Penguin.
Bowlby, J. (1988) *A Secure Base*. London: Routledge.
de Swaan, A. (1990) *The Management of Normality*. London: Routledge.
Feltham, C. (ed.) (1997) *Which Psychotherapy? Leading Exponents Explain Their Differences*. London: SAGE Publications.
Goldberg, D. and Huxley, P. (1992) *Common Mental Disorders: a Bio-social Model*. London: Routledge.
Guntrip, H. (1961) *Personality Structure and Human Interaction*. London: Hogarth Press.
Noyes, R. and Hoehn-Saric, R. (1998) *The Anxiety Disorders*. Cambridge: Cambridge University Press.

— Personality Disorders —

***Definition:* Personality disorders are psychiatric diagnoses which refer to disturbances in conduct. These enduring disturbances are associated with distress and recurrent interpersonal dysfunction in the person's life.**

Key points: *• The psychiatric classification of personality disorders is outlined • Criticisms of the use of the diagnosis of personality disorder are described.*

The origins of psychiatric interest, in what are now described as personality disorders, was limited to those who were deemed sane but who showed an absence of conscience and a lack of consideration for the rights of others. Today, this type of description would be limited only to what is called 'anti-social personality disorder' under *DSM-IV* and 'dissocial personality disorder' under *ICD-10*.

Even this older anti-social focus (what was called 'moral insanity') does not find a ready current consensus. For example the most extensive work in the area has been by a clinical psychologist, Robert Hare, who uses the term 'psychopathic disorder' to describe people with mixed features of anti-social, histrionic and narcissistic personality disorders. The term 'psychopathic disorder' is also used as a legal term in Britain to describe 'a persistent disorder or disability of mind (whether or not including subnormality of intelligence) which results in abnormally aggressive or seriously irresponsible conduct on the part of the patient and requires or is susceptible to medical treatment'.

The following types of personality disorder can be found in both *ICD-10* and *DSM*-IV, with some main diagnostic features being given in brackets:

- Paranoid (suspicious, mistrustful, resentful, grudge-bearing, jealous, self-important);
- Schizoid (emotionally cold, detached, aloof, lacking enjoyment, introspective);
- Schizotypal (socially anxious, eccentric, oddities of thought and perception);
- Borderline/emotionally unstable (chronic feelings of emptiness and fear of abandonment, recurrently suicidal and self-harming, unstable mood states);
- Dissocial/anti-social (callous to others, impulsive, lack of guilt and remorse, irresponsible, failure to take responsibility for actions);
- Anankastic/obsessive-compulsive (perfectionist, preoccupied by rules and details, over-conscientious, rigid and stubborn, pedantic, overly conventional);
- Histrionic (self-dramatizing, shallow, attention seeking, over-concern with physical attractiveness, suggestible);
- Anxious avoidant (fearful avoidance of others, fear of being criticized or humiliated);
- Dependent (compliant, lets others take responsibility, fear of being left to care for self, needs excessive help from others to make decisions).

In addition to this common list, narcissistic personality disorder appears in *DSM* but not *ICD*. It refers to these personal features: self-importance; grandiose ambitions about success or power; need for constant admiration; exploitative of others; arrogant and lacking in empathy. It may be noticed that self-centredness in its various forms is described in several types, not just narcissistic personality disorder.

There are a number of criticisms that can be levelled at the concept of personality disorder and, by implication, any of its types. These criticisms can be summarized by the following questions.

- *What is personality?* While most psychologists still use this term to describe a person's enduring or stable character, not all embrace it. For example, the study of context-dependent identities has become more and more important for some psychologists. For those who subscribe in principle to the concept of personality there is a consensus, for now, that individuals can be described by the unique combination of points on five dimensions (openness to experience, conscientiousness, extraversion, agreeableness and neuroticism);
- *If personality is a unique blend of points on five continua, can a* category *of personality disorder be identified?* This highlights a problem for any system of diagnosis which operates with the digital rule of present/absent or ordered/disordered. The compromise is to agree on a quantifiable cut off on a dimension (an analog decision). An example of this is the medical definition of hypertension being a persistent diastolic blood pressure of over 95 or 100. The total absence of measured blood pressure is a symptom of being dead and so blood pressure can only be described meaningfully for live subjects on a continuum rather than as a category. Similarly, personality is a description of live subjects and so has to be described in relative rather than categorical terms. If personality disorder were defined by personality characteristics, a computation of five different scores on the personality dimensions would need to be measured. Currently, the diagnosis is not made using this method and no professional agreement exists on this method of case identification;
- *Can personality disorder be distinguished from other forms of mental disorder?* For any diagnosis to be valid it should be coherent and separate from other conditions. *ICD* explicitly distinguishes personality disorder from mental illness. However, earlier authorities on personality problems and insanity (such as Henderson and Cleckley) saw an overlap between the two or a connecting continuum. Turning to neurosis, types such as 'anxious avoidant', 'dependent', 'histrionic' and 'obsessive-compulsive' personality disorder are basically descriptions of *chronic* neurotic symptom presentation. Not only are these types of personality disorder not *distinguishable* from neurosis, they are fundamentally *constituted* by it;
- *Is the diagnosis of personality disorder used consistently?* This is known as the problem of reliability of diagnosis, which takes two forms.

Inter-rater reliability is checking whether different professionals agree on the diagnosis of the same patient. Test-retest reliability is checking whether the patient is diagnosed consistently over time. This is more important in the diagnosis of personality disorder than of illness, because the latter may change with remission or recovery. Because personality disorder is about enduring personal qualities then we would expect stability of scores. Reasonable test-retest reliability is found for anti-social, paranoid and borderline personality disorders but all of the other types have poor reliability;

- *Can personality disorder be readily differentiated from normality?* The problem this question highlights is that the qualities described as 'personality disordered' may lead to good social adjustment or significant success in some social contexts. The aggressive propensities of the psychopath may be expressed lucratively in a professional boxer or honourably in a soldier. The tedious, self-dramatizing attention seeking of a histrionic personality might find fame and fortune on the stage. An obsessive-compulsive personality might function very well and efficiently in an occupation which requires close and consistent attention to detail. A narcissist might find an esteemed career in political life or success in the leadership of a large organization. Moreover there are cultural and sub-cultural norms in which symptoms of personality disorder might blend. The passivity and dependency of some Asian and Arctic cultures may mirror many of the symptoms of dependent personality disorder. The dramatic and flamboyant norms of Mediterranean countries may mirror many of the symptoms of histrionic personality disorder;
- *Can the aetiology of personality disorder be specified?* This is easy to answer – 'no'. The validity of a medical diagnosis requires a clear aetiology. However, personality disorder shares this vulnerability with the diagnosis of functional mental illness. All functional diagnoses are defined in a circular way, rather than by aetiology. The diagnosis is made on the basis of symptoms and the symptoms are accounted for by the diagnosis:

  Q: why does this man molest children?
  A: because he is a psychopath.
  Q: how do we know that he is a psychopath?
  A: because he molests children;

- *Can personality disorder be treated?* This awkward question is both a legal and medical one. The definition of psychopathic disorder under current British law requires 'treatability'. Because it is about disordered personalities and personality is defined by stability of character, it also means that character is incorrigible in those who act in an anti-social manner. If a person's incorrigible conduct is deemed untreatable then, arguably, they must remain outside of psychiatric jurisdiction (a point that some psychiatrists often make to avoid responsibility for some patients). Treatment regimes for personality disorder either focus on mitigating the excesses of personal distress and dysfunction (as in the treatment of borderline personality disorder) or on reducing specific offending behaviours (as in the treatment of sex offenders, who might warrant a diagnosis of anti-social personality disorder). In other words, at best some of the *symptoms or behavioural features* of personality disorder may be treatable but not the disorder itself.

A final point to make about personality disorder is that it is basically a medical codification of people who recurrently act in a way that others disapprove of, condemn or find tiresome. The diagnosis is a way of expressing dislike, disgust or contempt for others. The term 'moral insanity' has resonances today. The diagnosis of personality disorder is still about moral attributions.

See also: *psychiatric diagnosis; forensic mental health services; creativity; fear.*

FURTHER READING

Alarcon, R.D. and Foulks, E.F. (1995) 'Personality disorders and culture: contemporary clinical views', *Cultural Diversity and Mental Health*, 1 (1): 3–17.

Blackburn, R. (1988) 'On moral judgements and personality disorders: the myth of psychopathic disorder re-visited', *British Journal of Psychiatry*, 153: 505–12.

Cleckley, H. (1941) *The Mask of Sanity*. St Louis, MS: C.V. Mosby.

Dolan, B. and Coid, J. (1993) *Psychopathic and Anti-social Personality Disorders: Treatment and Research Issues*. London: Gaskell.

Hare, R.D. (1993) *Without Conscience: the Disturbing World of the Psychopaths Among Us*. New York: Pocket.

Henderson, D.K. (1938) *Psychopathic States*. London: Wiley.

Linehan, M.M. (1993) *Cognitive Behaviour Therapy of Borderline Personality Disorder*. New York: Guilford Press.

Livesley, J.W. (ed.) (1995) *The DSM-IV Personality Disorders*. New York: Guilford Press.

Pilgrim, D. (2001) 'Disordered personalities and disordered concepts', *Journal of Mental Health*, 10 (3): 253–66.

Substance Misuse

***Definition:* The use of a psychoactive substance in a way that causes harm to self or others.**

Key points: *• Substance misuse is described, mainly using alcohol abuse as an example • The public health, as well as individual consequences of substance misuse are discussed.*

Psychiatrists consider substance misuse to be both a free-standing mental disorder and a common presenting problem in medicine, affecting health in a variety of ways. The diagnosis appears in both the *International Classification of Diseases* (World Health Organization, 1992) and the *Diagnostic and Statistical Manual of Mental Disorders (DSM)* (American Psychiatric Association, 1994).

Because of the prevalent use of alcohol, it is considered to be a major public health problem and so will be the main exemplar in this chapter. Excessive alcohol use has a demonstrable influence on both the health status of its users and on third parties affected by intoxicated behaviour. For example, excessive and prolonged alcohol consumption increases the chances of heart disease, neurological degeneration and some forms of cancer. It is specifically linked to premature death from cirrhosis of the liver. Suicidal behaviour and depressed mood, as well as job loss, are also linked to alcohol intoxication. At the same time, and arguably of greater importance because there may be multiple innocent victims, substance misuse increases the probability of road traffic accidents, domestic violence, child neglect, sexual offending and violent assaults on strangers.

The health effects related to self and others of lesser used drugs are more complicated. For example, the use of heroin and its prescribed medical substitute methadone increase the risk of road traffic accidents but do not seem to be linked strongly to violence against others. Non-violent acquisitive crime and prostitution are linked though to heroin use because of the drug's high financial cost to the user. By contrast, crack cocaine is strongly linked to violent action.

The risk associated with the opioids (drugs synthesized to chemically mimic, or ones derived directly from, opium) is complicated by the way that they are used. The unsafe, illegal supply of heroin and its common intravenous method of administration create particular and often lethal hazards. These include accidental over-dosing, because drug purity in local supplies varies, and acquired infections, such as HIV and hepatitis. Intravenous use is preferred because of the 'rush' of euphoria it creates in the recipient. This is one reason why addicts are less keen on the oral use of methadone, which prevents distressing heroin withdrawal symptoms but provides no 'rush' prior to a comforting and prolonged heroin stupor ('nodding').

For those who consider substance misuse to be a diagnosable psychiatric condition rather than a bad habit, injurious to self and others, then *ICD* and *DSM* are at hand. Both classificatory systems specify the following substances implicated in the diagnosis: alcohol, caffeine, cannabis, cocaine, hallucinogens, solvents (or inhalants), nicotine (or tobacco), opioids, and sedatives and hypnotics. Amphetamines and phencyclidine, an obsolete anaesthetic used as a recreational drug in the US but rarely in the UK, are included in *DSM* but not in *ICD*. Amphetamine-like substances, such as MDMA ('ecstasy'), may be specified in new editions of *ICD* and *DSM*.

The criteria used for the diagnosis in *DSM* are more elaborate than in *ICD*. The latter simply refers to 'a pattern of psychoactive substance use that is causing damage to health; the damage may be to physical or mental health'. The *DSM* list is longer and refers to a list of one or more of the following 'clinically significant impairments' over a 12-month period manifested in: failures in role obligations in work, school or home; substance use in situations of physical hazard; legal problems; and persistent inter-personal problems linked to the use. This stipulation of a 12-month defining period would exclude the public health implications of those who, when acutely intoxicated, episodically or on a one-off basis, might cause serious harm to others.

When it comes to defining dependency or dependence, both systems emphasize: a compulsion to use the drug; a tendency to increase dose levels because of tolerance; withdrawal effects; a persistent focus on the use of the drug to the detriment or exclusion of other activities; and a failure to control the habit, despite feedback about its consequences. It is clear that some of the substances listed in *DSM* and *ICD* are not dependency forming but are very psychoactive (e.g. the hallucinogens). Others are very dependency forming but barely psychoactive in the experience of the user, so only strong withdrawal effects are noted (e.g.

caffeine and nicotine). Sometimes 'dependence' is distinguished from 'addiction', with the presence of *physical* withdrawal effects indicating the latter and their absence suggesting the *psychological* nature of the former.

Estimates about the prevalence of substance misuse vary from place to place. North American studies of alcohol misuse indicate a one-year prevalence of 7–10%, with a lifetime risk of 14–20% (Regier et al., 1994). This compares with a one-year prevalence of 4.7% in the UK (Meltzer et al., 1994). Some of this difference could be accounted for by different methods of data collection (the US studies included homeless populations but the UK one did not). When homeless populations are sampled, then the prevalence rate of alcohol abuse rises to around 40% in Britain (Gill et al., 1996).

Also, the demographic pattern of problem drinking changes over time, as well as place. While cirrhosis levels have declined overall in recent years in Southern Europe, in Northern Europe excessive drinking has significantly increased in young females, indicating that women will increasingly become medical casualties of their habit with age. Given the recklessness linked to intoxication ('disinhibition'), this also means that female perpetrators of violence and other anti-social acts are tending to increase in number. Another indication of the social cost of alcohol consumption is its impact on hospital admission (in the UK this is around 10%, in both psychiatric and general medical admissions). Young binge drinking places a particular acute stress on both law enforcement and emergency medical services at weekends.

Because substance misuse occurs typically in people who are deemed to be sane, health professionals may hold an ambivalent attitude towards patients, similar to that about those with a diagnosis of personality disorder. Indeed sometimes persistent multiple drug use and its behavioural consequences are used to diagnose anti-social personality disorder. Because of the strong moral discourse surrounding drug use, a tension exists between traditional medical paternalism, in which the patient is treated sympathetically as the victim of an affliction, and the cultural norm (which health workers are embedded in and so reflect) of condemning the user and morally exhorting them to change for the better. This ambivalence also appears in the treatment programmes offered. These all require personal commitment and honesty from the user and so it is often difficult to separate medical descriptions of cure or recovery from common sense ones of moral reform.

A particular point about substance misuse is its role in the debate about violence and mental disorder. Psychotic patients who abuse substances are more dangerous than others in the general population. However, those who do not abuse substances are not more dangerous. Moreover, substance misuse *alone* leads to a significant increase in the risk of danger to self or others. This is important because if substance misuse is formally within the jurisdiction of psychiatry, then users become psychiatric patients and raise the profile of violence in this particular population. It also skews our association of suicide with mental health problems. Suicidal behaviour is correlated with mental health problems but by no means limited to them.

If substance misuse were not framed as a psychiatric problem (but, say, a social or moral one) then a sub-group of violent and suicidal intoxicated people would be removed from the 'dangerous to self or others' component of psychiatric populations. This might then beg a question about whether the State should intervene to alter substance misuse and, if so, what alternative interventions and view of the problem would replace those associated with 'psychiatric treatment' and medical paternalism. A bridge between a psychiatric approach and that used within a lay view of morality is the widespread and sustained success of the organization *Alcoholics Anonymous (AA)* which began in 1935 and continues to operate globally. It emphasizes personal responsibility for recovery but starts with a confession that the person is powerless in the face of the drug and that life has become unmanageable.

AA has become a prototype self-help model for a range of addictive problems and so we now also see, for example, *Narcotics Anonymous*, *Sex Addicts Anonymous*, *Gamblers Anonymous* and *Overeaters Anonymous*. These self-help initiatives also point up the tendency for *any* compulsive habit (from cigarette smoking and shopping to sexual promiscuity and shoplifting) to be thought of as a psychiatric problem. Also, the ambiguous word 'compulsive' here indicates that some people are compelled to break rules (in the case of this section, rules of sobriety, moderation and decorum) and others are compelled to comply with them (in the case of the overly conformist obsessive-compulsive personality disorder). The abstinence model of AA may suggest that people are exhorted and supported to move from one end to the other of a compulsive continuum.

The widespread contemporary societal preoccupation with a range of addictive behaviours throws into relief our modern struggle with the use and abuse of individual freedom. The wide inclusion of so many addictions reflects recent forms of social organization based upon consumption, with the latter shaping identities and modern definitions of both normality and pathology (Reith, 2004).

An argument for retaining a medical view of substance misuse is the good evidence that it is a form of self-medication to reduce stress or to improve mood (even if these personal short-term strategies may be counter-productive in the long term). However, analysts of the role of substance use in the self-management of experienced stress point out that many do not progress to fulfil criteria for a psychiatric disorder (Aneshensel, 1999). Put differently, beneath the lifetime risk of 14–20% for alcohol misuse, noted earlier, lies a large number of people (probably most of the remaining 80%+) who use alcohol moderately, or excessively on occasions, to release tension or to improve their mood. This point obviously applies less in those countries where alcohol use is illegal or is culturally constrained.

See also: *personality disorders; risks to and from people with mental health problems.*

REFERENCES

American Psychiatric Association (1994) *Diagnostic and Statistical Manual of Mental Disorders (Fourth Edition)*. Washington: American Psychiatric Association.

Aneshensel, C.S. (1999) 'Outcomes of the stress process', in A.V. Horwitz and T.L. Scheid (eds), *A Handbook for the Study of Mental Health*. Cambridge: Cambridge University Press.

Gill, B., Meltzer, H., Hinds, K. and Pettigrew, M. (1996) *Psychiatric Morbidity Among Homeless People. OPCS Surveys of Psychiatric Morbidity in Great Britain*. London: HMSO.

Meltzer, H., Gill, B. and Pettigrew, M. (1994) *The Prevalence of Psychiatric Morbidity Among Adults Aged 16–64 Living in Private Households. OPCS Surveys of Psychiatric Morbidity in Great Britain*. London: HMSO.

Regier, D.A., Narrow, W.E., Rae, D.S., Manderscheld, R.W., Locke, B.Z. and Goodwin, F.K. (1994) 'The *de facto* US mental and addictive disorders service', *Archives of General Psychiatry*, 50: 85–94.

Reith, G. (2004) 'Consumption and its discontents: addiction, identity and the problem of freedom', *British Journal of Sociology*, 55 (2): 283–98.

World Health Organization (1992) *The ICD-10 Classification of Mental and Behavioural Disorders*. Geneva: WHO.

— Learning Disability —

***Definition:* The term 'learning disability' is used currently to describe people of low intelligence who are impaired in their social competence. It is also used to describe both the services for these people and a sub-specialty of psychiatry. Terms used previously include: 'learning difficulties', 'mental handicap', 'mental retardation', 'mental subnormality', 'mental deficiency' and 'idiocy'. Current variations on the term include: 'people with learning disabilities' and 'learning disabled people'.**

Key points: *• The history of learning disability and its links to psychiatric services are described • The shift from a medical to a social model of learning disability is outlined.*

At the start of the nineteenth century, with the mass segregation of a range of deviant populations in hospitals, asylums, workhouses and 'colonies', those with learning disabilities and those with mental health problems could be found together. The Lunacy Act of 1845 stipulated that 'idiots, lunatics or persons of unsound mind' should be certified and detained in asylums (Saunders, 1985). A distinction was made by the end of the century between two forms of intellectual impairment: 'idiocy', manifest from infancy and 'dementia', developing later in life. In Britain, as in the rest of Europe and North America, the gradual legislative division of 'idiocy' from 'lunacy' became apparent. For example, the 1890 Lunacy Act, emerged separately from the 1886 Idiots Act.

This separation was maintained in the subsequent 1913 Mental Deficiency Act and the 1930 Mental Treatment Act. However, some legal ambiguity remains. For example, current mental health legislation, covering mentally disordered offenders, includes 'mental impairment' and 'severe mental impairment'. These refer to people with learning disabilities who are considered to be a grave and immediate danger to others. Some of them are detained in *mental health* facilities, such as the high security Rampton Hospital. Medium secure facilities for others are dotted around the country.

The prejudicial lay notion has long existed that mental health problems and learning disabilities are the same type of mental incapacity, disorder or disability. This amalgam prejudice cuts both ways. In ordinary language, all those with mental health problems might inaccurately be considered to be 'stupid' and those with learning problems might all wrongly be considered to be 'mad'. In English-speaking countries both groups might be dismissed as being 'mental', in a pejorative or scoffing way, by others.

At the turn of the twentieth century, this conflation of the two groups in the lay mentality was mirrored, to a degree, in the professional domain, as psychiatrists took over the jurisdiction of intellectual impairment in mental handicap hospitals, not just the management of madness in mental hospitals. A legacy of this today is that learning disability is a sub-speciality of psychiatry.

At times, professionals and relatives of patients have episodically made painstaking attempts to point out that the client's problems in each are quite different. However, this understandable attempt to put a conceptual distance between the two groups of patients is itself problematic. It may imply that someone with a learning disability is in some way immune from mental health problems. This is both logically and empirically untenable. People with learning disabilities, like anyone else, can develop mental health problems. Also, on average, those with a diagnosis of schizophrenia have a lower intelligence than the measured norm (using the tradition of the tested intelligence quotient or IQ). They also usually manifest social impairments. Psychiatrists may see this as evidence of schizophrenia being a neuro-developmental disorder. (However, the *upper range* of IQs in those with a diagnosis of schizophrenia is the same as the general population.)

In the light of the above problems about overlapping psychological characteristics, attempts to keep the two types of patient groups separate may have had the perverse effect of disenfranchising those with learning disabilities, as their access to mental health provision is restricted. On the other hand, some psychotic patients may have unrecognized learning difficulties. Thus, those with both learning disabilities *and* mental health problems can 'fall between two stools' of service provision.

Because learning disability is defined by poor cognitive capacity, judged by the presence of both a low IQ and impaired social competence, then medical jurisdiction can be queried. People with learning disabilities overwhelmingly have training, educational and social, rather than medical, needs. However, for the time being, people with learning disabilities and their families are largely cared for by the same occupational mix as those with mental health problems. The training of these psychiatrists, nurses and psychologists overlaps with, but is also different from, that of their colleagues working in mental health services. While some learning disability services have now shifted from the NHS to social service jurisdiction, the professionals working in them are still predominantly trained in a health service context.

The retention of learning disability in medicalized settings can be justified partially by a large core group of patients with genetic abnormalities (such as Down's Syndrome) or a range of congenital metabolic abnormalities. Also, some post-natal acquired brain damage has an explicit neurological aetiology. The latter may include head injury, malnutrition, lead poisoning or brain infection. These inherited, congenital and post-natal medical histories can lead to a learning disability emerging during childhood and provide fair grounds for framing them as true medical neurology cases. Some of these infants have very short lives and so do not become adults with a learning disability (for example, in those with Tay-Sachs Disease and Hurler's Syndrome).

This leaves an ambiguous or marginal role for psychiatry (rather than neurology or psychology). Even if there is a known biological cause for the patients' learning disabilities, their behavioural problems require social and psychological responses. This is similar to the position of older people with dementia, where biological aetiology is proven or is likely but psycho-social interventions (especially with family members) are mainly implicated. As with much of the work of psychiatry, biological aetiology (known or assumed) does not always lead to appropriate, acceptable or effective biological treatments. For example, the use of major tranquillizers ('anti-psychotics') in learning disability treatment has been controversial. At the same time, the more appropriate use of psychological techniques, preferred by clinical psychologists, to deal with violent or challenging behaviour of patients is not without controversy (McDonnell and Sturmey, 1993).

Moves towards the de-medicalization of learning disability and towards a social model of understanding and provision have come on three fronts: first, most of the old 'mental handicap' hospitals have now been closed down and their residents shifted to small community-based living facilities. Some of the challenging or dysfunctional problems of residents in large institutions were a result of social isolation and a lack of meaningful daily activity ('institutionalization'). However, since patients have moved into the community, many of these problems are still reported, indicating that expectations about the benefits of simply resettling patients may have been over-optimistic.

Second, the demand for more human rights for people with learning disabilities arose in the 1970s, with the professionally driven 'normalization' movement (Nirje, 1970; Wolfensberger, 1972). Normalization demands that devalued people have their right to a normal existence restored as much as possible. The campaign to educate children with learning disabilities in ordinary schools is a practical manifestation of this normalization ideology.

Third, a new social movement of learning disabled people has campaigned for their increasing rights as citizens. This user-led but advocate-supported movement has reinforced the work on citizenship demands started by the normalization movement. This parallels the emphasis on social inclusion demanded by people with mental health problems.

Returning to the development of mental health problems in those who are learning disabled, a paradox exists. On the one hand the prevalence of some mental health problems is considered to be higher than in non-learning disabled populations. On the other hand, the ability to detect psychiatric disorders is confounded by communication difficulties. The higher rate of psychotic disorders in learning disabled populations compared to the general population reinforces the psychiatric assumption that 'schizophrenia' is a neurodevelopmental disorder.

Mood disorders are diagnosed less often in people with learning disabilities. Estimates of diagnosable personality disorder in those with learning disabilities in the community are as high as 30%, with a further 20% being described as having 'abnormalities of personality' (Khan et al., 1997). Also, anxiety may be expressed differently in this group of patients. The communication problems people with a learning disability have when representing themselves to others suggest that an effective and helpful response to those who also have mental health problems requires particular professional skills and good inter-disciplinary collaboration (Drotar and Sturm, 1996).

See also: *mental health; stigma; social exclusion; personality disorders.*

REFERENCES

Drotar, D.D. and Sturm, L.A. (1996) 'Interdisciplinary collaboration in the practice of mental retardation', in J.W. Jacobson and J.A. Mullick (eds), *Manual of Diagnosis and Professional Practice in Mental Retardation*. Washington: American Psychiatric Association.

Khan, A., Cowan, C. and Roy, A. (1997) 'Personality disorders in people with learning disabilities: a community survey', *Journal of Intellectual Disability Research*, 41: 324–30.

McDonnell, A.A. and Sturmey, P. (1993) 'Managing violent and aggressive behaviour: towards better practice', in R.S.P. Jones and C. Eayrs (eds), *Challenging Behaviours and People with Learning Disabilities: a Psychological Perspective*. Kidderminster: British Institute of Learning Disabilities.

Nirje, B. (1970) 'Normalization', *Journal of Mental Subnormality*, 31: 62–70.

Saunders, J. (1985) 'Quarantining the weak-minded; psychiatric definitions of degeneracy and the late Victorian asylum', in W.F. Bynum, R. Porter and M. Shepherd (eds), *The Anatomy of Madness (Volume III)*. London: Tavistock.

Wolfensberger, W. (1972) *The Principle of Normalisation in Human Services*. Toronto: National Institute of Mental Retardation.

Causes and Constructs

***Definition:* Causal statements are empirical claims which trace a current condition to one or more factors in the past. Knowledge claims about constructs refer, in this case, to the ways in which 'mental disorder' or 'mental health' are conceptualized or represented. These claims do not reflect empirical research but pre-empirical or non-empirical inquiries about the way in which mental states are defined and socially negotiated.**

Key points: • *Biological, psychological and social explanations for mental disorder are summarized* • *The conceptual problems of psychiatric knowledge are discussed.*

Knowledge claims about the causes of a particular mental state refer to the proven or assumed antecedent factors that brought it into being. If a mental disorder is being considered this is called its 'aetiology'. If a state of mental well-being is being considered, it is called its 'salotogenesis'.

The study of mental health and mental disorders, as in other fields of inquiry, is complicated. It is particularly problematic for two main reasons. First there is much disagreement about whether mental health and mental disorder are *meaningful* concepts. 'Mental illnesses' and 'personality disorders', in particular, have been subjected to particular criticism in relation to their legitimacy, validity or meaningfulness. Second, even when there *is* agreement about defining the general and particular nature of mental health and mental disorder, there are large disagreements about the cause or causes implicated.

Given these two serious considerations about the study of the scope of this book, it is probably wise for any student of mental health (whether new to it or not) to proceed with caution. However, often professional or economic interests lead to strong and definitive claims in a field when humility and tentative inquiry are usually advised. To illustrate this here are some summary points about this contested field:

- *Bio-determinism* Since the middle of the nineteenth century most psychiatrists have argued that severe mental illness is caused by a genetically programmed disease of the brain, even though there still remains no firm empirical evidence to support this claim. Mental illnesses 'run in families' but obey no simple genetic rules. The very fact that these claims can be found at their strongest in relation to functional mental illnesses, such as 'schizophrenia', illustrates that professional interests rather than disinterested empirical inquiry have shaped discussions about causation. Bio-determinism is both a mainstream orthodoxy and a focus of controversy, as it is traceable to a eugenic tradition. Its current strong advocates include the North American psychiatrist Samuel Guze;
- *Psychological determinism* Some psychiatrists and most psychologists have emphasized the psychological antecedents of mental disorder. However, there is much disagreement about what psychological causes mean. Different psychological researchers and therapists have emphasized: intra-psychic conflict, attachment problems, trauma, operant and classical conditioning, distorted cognitions and existential challenges. Many psychiatrists who are bio-determinists about psychotic conditions will consider the central role of some form of psychological determinism in neurotic presentations. This has led at times to a division of labour in mental health services between psychiatry and psychology, with the former mainly dealing with psychosis and the latter neurosis;
- *Social determinism* Some mental health researchers from different

backgrounds (psychiatry, psychology and sociology) have argued that social antecedents are the most important to trace because they can point to policy interventions to improve mental health. This interdisciplinary field is usually called 'social psychiatry'. Many in this field argue that individuals may have a susceptibility to a disorder but that social factors precipitate and maintain it. The susceptibility may be derived from biological psychological or social factors in the past, which prompts the next position;

- *Biopsychosocial determinism* An integrated or eclectic position described at the end of the last point is championed by those operating a biopsychosocial model. This model does not challenge the basic validity of psychiatric diagnosis but does argue that the patient's particular biographical picture should be privileged, when understanding why they are presenting with these particular symptoms at this time in their life. Thus the emphasis in the model is upon multi-factorial aetiology and patient-centredness. The origins of the model can be traced to the work of the Swiss psychiatrist Adolf Meyer, who used the term 'psychobiology' in the early twentieth century.

It can be pointed out that these competing theories about the causes of mental disorder are also reflected when mental health is being understood. But because the latter remains less investigated and psychiatry has been such a contested field, mental disorder is the focus here.

Moving now to the constructs of mental disorder or mental health, these refer to the ways in which they are conceptualized or represented. They can be investigated using three methods:

- *Conceptual analysis* This is favoured by philosophical realists who are critical or sceptical about empirical claims in science. They look closely at the coherence of the concepts at the centre of an investigation. For example, if a claim is being made about the cause or causes of 'schizophrenia' the conceptual validity of the latter is analysed in detail;
- *Frame analysis* This does not challenge the notion of causes but examines the way in which a problem comes to be socially negotiated by parties in interaction. Frame analysis was promoted by labelling theorists like Erving Goffman;
- *Deconstruction* This methodology is linked to various forms of social constructivism. It shares the concerns about the social

negotiation of reality with frame analysis but may go further in two senses. First, it asks questions about the interests being served by problems being theorized in this or that way. Why is biodeterminism elaborated to the exclusion of other explanations by the psychiatric profession and the drug companies? Why do psychologists want to privilege psychological determinism? Why is this mental health problem being researched in this way at this point in time in this particular society? Second, it may challenge the notion of causes in principle. This more radical position, associated with the philosopher Michel Foucault, argues that reality cannot be defined independently of the ideas and practices that represent or embody it ('discursive practices'). While labelling theorists might favour frame analysis to problematize secondary deviance, radical constructivists question psychiatric knowledge itself (representations of primary deviance).

See also: *labelling theory; psychiatric diagnosis; the 'myth of mental illness'; eugenics.*

FURTHER READING

Bolton, D. and Hill, J. (1996) *Mind, Meaning and Mental Disorder: the Nature of Causal Explanations in Psychology and Psychiatry*. Oxford: Oxford University Press.

Castle, D.J. (2004) 'Improving lives: the balance between biology and psychosocial interventions research for the functional psychoses?', *Journal of Mental Health*, 13 (3): 229–34.

Goffman, E. (1974) *Frame Analysis*. New York: Harper & Row.

Guze, S. (1989) 'Biological psychiatry: is there any other kind?', *Psychological Medicine*, 19: 315–23.

Miller, P. and Rose, N. (eds) (1985) *The Power of Psychiatry*. Oxford: Polity.

Parker, I., Georgaca, E., Harper, D., McLaughlin, T. and Stowell-Smith, M. (1995) *Deconstructing Psychopathology*. London: SAGE Publications.

Pilgrim, D. (2002) 'The biopsychosocial model in Anglo-American psychiatry: past, present and future?', *Journal of Mental Health*, 11 (6): 585–94.

Tyrer, P. and Sternberg, D. (1987) *Models for Mental Disorder*. Chichester: Wiley.

Physical Health

Definition: *In its simplest terms physical health refers to soundness of the body. It is often defined negatively, though, by the absence of disease. A person may be healthy but not necessarily fit. The latter implies a readiness to maintain health and the body being at its maximum potential.*

Key points: *• The inter-play between physical and mental health is discussed and examples given • Cautions about the notion of 'somatization' are rehearsed.*

This entry appears in a book on mental health for two reasons. First, a person's physical health status predicts their mental health status and vice versa. For example, psychiatric patients have high rates of physical morbidity. They are four times more likely to die of cardio-vascular and respiratory disease and five times more at risk of becoming diabetic. Second, some abnormalities of the body (particularly of the nervous system) lead to psychological, as well as physical, symptoms. The separation of mind and body is called 'Cartesian dualism' by philosophers, following the trend begun by Descartes of discussing them separately. In some cultures this dualism does not exist, which is reflected in the way words are used to describe health and illness.

The inter-play of physical and mental health has led to a group of mental health professionals ('liaison psychiatrists' and 'clinical health psychologists') working in areas of physical medicine and surgery. A number of points can be summarized about the enmeshment of physical and mental health:

- *Psychosomatic illnesses* These are physical illnesses in which psychological functioning makes a causal contribution. For example, gastro-intestinal disturbances in an anxious person may lead to chronic dyspepsia or ulceration of the stomach or gut. At one time, ulcers of this sort were thought of, overwhelmingly, as being of psychological origin but, more recently, bacterial causes have also been identified;

- *Psychogenic disorders* This is a more general term, which includes psychosomatic illnesses and other conditions in which minor symptoms of illness are exaggerated in a distressed fashion by the patient ('hypochondriasis' or 'hypochondriacal overlay') or the person has dramatic symptoms with no apparent physical evidence of cause ('hysterical conversion disorders'). Even more dramatically some people inflict harm on themselves to receive emergency medical treatment ('Munchausen's Syndrome'). In very rare cases, an extension of this are parents or care staff who harm children to seek medical attention ('Munchausen's Syndrome-by-Proxy'). Psychiatrists use the term 'somatization' to describe the expression of psychological distress in bodily terms;
- *Somato-psychological reactions* This is when a physical disease or acquired disability leads to psychological distress. An example of this is the way in which people differ in their psychological adaptation to losing, or losing the use of, limbs. Some people develop a prolonged grief reaction to the loss or their personality becomes irritable, whereas others do not react in these ways;
- *Neurological diseases* These invariably have psychological consequences. In dementia the person becomes disorientated in time and space and short-term memory problems are evident. Amnesia predominates in those who chronically abuse alcohol and these patients may also experience visual hallucinations ('Korsakoff's Psychosis'). As another example of the mutual influence of mind and body, cardio-vascular functioning can be affected negatively by chronic stress and behavioural factors, such as poor diet and a low exercise lifestyle. In turn, these effects can create chronic hypertension, which increases the risk of dementia – a neurological disease;
- *Drug reactions and withdrawal* Some drugs create temporary psychological effects. This largely describes the effects of psychoactive drugs like caffeine, heroin, benzodiazepines and hallucinogens. Occasionally, psychotic reactions occur in the wake of amphetamine and cannabis use. Some prescribed medications for physical illness have behavioural effects (for example, some oral anti-histamines can cause sedation and an increased risk of accidents). Drug withdrawal also has psychological consequences. For example, nicotine withdrawal produces agitation in the smoker;
- *The psychological benefits of physical exercise* Physical exercise creates mental health gain for two reasons. First it creates changes in the biochemical functioning of the brain to raise mood. Second, the sense of control, which exercise bestows, raises self-esteem. For these reasons

physical exercise can be used successfully in the treatment of 'mild to moderate' presentations of generalized anxiety and depression;

- *The psychological impact of multiple illness* This is particularly relevant in older people because the probability of multiple illness increases with age, but it could apply at any age in an individual case. Multiple illness creates pain and pain is demoralizing. It also creates functional deficits (around movement and access to routine daily activities). The latters create a sense of loss and loss of control in the patient, which is saddening for them;
- *The ambiguity of pain* Neuroscientists studying pain note that it has sensory, cognitive and emotional aspects (experienced concurrently by the patient in a 'pain matrix'). The traditional distinction between physical and psychological pain is that the latter has no obvious sensory source (such as a tumour, scald or wound). However, experientially, some very depressed patients describe a form of physical pain and they may have very strong beliefs about their body being diseased. Also, some forms of illness such as fybromyalgia and irritable bowel syndrome, which include a dominant symptom of acute pain, are correlated with distressing psychological histories (of trauma or abuse). Again this highlights the ambiguities surrounding the experience of distress in a social context, which maintains the Cartesian split between mind and body;
- *The physical correction of healthy bodies for intended mental health gain* This is contentious in relation to both the behaviour of professionals and their patients. On the one hand under *DSM-IV*, patients who complain unreasonably that some part of their anatomy requires correction are diagnosed as suffering from 'body dysmorphic disorder'. On the other hand, cosmetic surgeons are kept in business by the needs of patients, with no obvious disease, demanding and acquiring corrective intervention, such as face lifts and breast enlargement. Another example in this controversial area is the intervention of surgeons, physicians and psychiatrists in the treatment of transsexualism. Outside of the domain of sex-change negotiations between lay people and professionals, body modification is also common now in a range of unilateral decisions made by adult citizens – body piercing, tattooing and scarification. All of these activities are aimed, among other things, at some form of mental health gain via individual expression, group identity and resistance to conformity.

Some controversies arise from the above points. In relation to the last one, surgical intervention to alter appearance raises ethical and political questions about the mutilation of healthy tissue and the use of scarce health service resources for people whose medical needs can be queried. The high rates of continued psychological distress after sex changes also point up the problem of assuming that transsexuals are always psychologically satisfied with a newly acquired gender status.

Psychogenic illnesses have also been surrounded by disputes. By definition, hypochondriacal patients are chronically disaffected with the medical profession. Under *DSM*, hypochondriasis is a 'somatoform disorder'. To the embarrassment of their treating psychiatrist, some patients with this label may transpire to have an unrecognized physical pathology. For this reason, the medical profession increasingly is using the more cautious description of 'medically unexplained symptoms'. Some other patients described as 'somatizers' have been involved in a collective opposition movement. An example is those with 'chronic fatigue syndrome', who sometimes resent their problems being ascribed to underlying psychological causes.

A final example of a controversy about the 'somatization' thesis is that in some cultures the presentation of physical illness has a different significance to that applying in the norms of Western medicine. For example, a common medical assumption is that South Asian patients, who are 'really' depressed, present with bodily complaints. This psychiatric tendency has not escaped without criticism.

See also: *functional and organic mental illnesses; psychiatric diagnosis; substance misuse.*

FURTHER READING

Banks, J. and Prior, L. (2001) 'Doing things with illness: the micro-politics of the CFS clinic', *British Journal of Sociology*, 52 (2): 11–23.

Fenton, S. and Sadiq-Sangster, A. (1996) 'Culture, relativism and mental distress', *Sociology of Health and Illness*, 18 (1): 66–85.

Guthrie, F. and Creed, F. (eds) (1996) *Liaison Psychiatry*. London: Gaskell.

MacLachlan, M. (1997) *Culture and Health*. London: Wiley.

Manu, P. (1998) *Functional Somatic Syndromes*. Cambridge: Cambridge University Press.

Pitts, V. (2003) *In the Flesh: the Cultural Politics of Body Modification*. New York: Palgrave.

Pleasure

***Definition:* 'A feeling of satisfaction or joy; sensuous enjoyment as an object of life' (The Concise Oxford Dictionary).**

Key points: • *The relevance of pleasure to the topic of mental health is examined with examples given • The importance of the denial of pleasure in religious and psychological systems of thought is discussed.*

Pleasure is not discussed at length in most of the literature of mental health professionals. The experience contains the fluid interplay of closely related emotions on the emotional circumplex (see the section on Sadness). These are at one end of the pleasant–unpleasant dimension and experienced subjectively as being: 'content', 'glad', 'pleased', 'happy', 'delighted' and 'excited'. In everyday language, pleasure implies a state of being – it is constituted by thought and action, not just a feeling state. The two aspects of the dictionary definition point to pleasure as both an emotion and a motivation or intention.

Despite the relative lack of discussion about it in the literature, pleasure-seeking does have implications for mental health in a number of ways:

- *The pursuit of pleasure is a civil right in modern democracies* In this sense, the achievement of pleasure could be seen as being close to the World Health Organization's definition of psychological well-being. Human behaviour includes a number of pleasure-seeking activities. If pursued with due caution, they can achieve temporary or recurrent happiness, buffer the person against mental health problems and create no long-term risk to the individual or others. Examples here would include satisfying work and sexual activity, moderate intoxication, telling jokes or listening to comedy, listening to or playing music, watching or playing sport, preparing or eating food, reading or writing, watching television, going to the theatre, walking and other exercise and so on. Some on this list might appear as virtuous hobbies at the end of a CV (others might be omitted). Freud defined work and love as the two touchstones of positive mental health. He emphasized the tension between the pleasure principle, our natural tendency to avoid pain, and its modification by the demands of civilization (the reality principle). The first was about infantile wish fulfilment, whereas the second was about adult adaptation. Other analysts, such as Wilhelm Reich, were more emphatic that free and pleasurable sexual expression was a prerequisite of avoiding both mental and physical health problems. His view was that pleasure was positive and healthy and Reich elevated erotic love to a special health-giving position. He argued that mandatory monogamy was an impediment to mental health but also that pornography and prostitution were oppressive and unhealthy expressions of sexual need;

- *Short-term access to a state of pleasure can lead to long-term mental health problems* The most obvious example of this is in relation to intoxication. As drunks with hangovers know, intoxication is a fleeting form of pleasure but also one that seductively re-engages the victim. Heroin addicts describe hours of intense warm pleasure after the initial 'rush' of an intra-venous injection. These transient experiences in those who misuse substances are so overwhelmingly addictive that they are sought repeatedly, often at the expense of all other social obligations or personal needs. Other examples of pleasure-as-danger include the risk of HIV infection in unguarded sexual activity and intra-venous drug use, and the risk of death or injury from fast driving;
- *Pleasure can be a precarious or absent state in some mental health problems* The clearest example of this is in relation to bi-polar disorder. However, the periods of exuberance, grandiosity, and industry in 'high' phases are not inevitably experienced as pleasurable – sometime patients express distress when they are manic. Also, unrestrained mania can lead to exhaustion and even death. The depressive collapse that ensues after a manic episode is certainly not a pleasurable state. The inability to experience pleasure may also be indicative of other problems like those with diagnoses of schizoid personality disorder and schizophrenia (where it is a 'negative symptom'). A lack of pleasure appears in psychiatric texts as 'loss of libido' or 'anhedonia';
- *Humanistic psychology takes a permissive view of pleasure* Examples of this can be found in the humanistic psychology literature of the 1960s (sometimes called the 'human potential' or 'growth' movement) and the more recent study of positive psychology. In the

first case, in reaction to the negative emphasis of psychoanalysis, which emphasized the abandonment of wish fulfilment and the need for the growing child to rescind its wishes, the 'growth movement' was permissive and positive. People were encouraged to elaborate and pursue their fantasies. However, the human potential movement was not merely hedonistic, as it also encouraged people to find meaning in all forms of experience, not just pleasure. In the case of positive psychology, there is an emphasis on the study of how people achieve and succeed, rather than on studying their defects. It studies the promotion of positive personal traits, such as inter-personal effectiveness and self determination. This is a recent elaboration of the work of American humanistic psychologists, such as Carl Rogers and Abraham Maslow. Positive psychology puts personal well-being at the centre of benign inter-personal processes of support and tolerance. The experience of pleasure in this view of mental health is not an end in itself but a permitted outcome or experience.

The notion that people should be able to achieve and sustain pleasure is at odds with some philosophical and scientific positions about the human condition (though hedonism has always had its philosophical advocates). For example, Buddhism and existentialism tend to emphasize suffering and angst as integral to the human condition and that striving against this truth is futile. Paradoxically, they also argue that pleasure may be achieved for periods of time by not striving for it.

The major deistic faiths tend to emphasize the denial of pleasure as a prerequisite of salvation or spiritual experience. For example, celibacy and frugality are emphasized in the Catholic Church, in its clergy and other religious members (nuns and monks). All Christian and Jewish groups demand that sexual pleasure is limited to monogamous relationships. Islam is less clear about the latter demand, as it sometimes tolerates polygamy, but it concurs with the other two faiths about the taboo on pre-marital and extra-marital sexual activity.

Most faiths restrict access to types of food and encourage periods of restraint and abstinence. Muslims and Mormons are not permitted alcohol and the latters are denied caffeine. Sexual abstinence and fasting are also associated with deeper spiritual understanding in Hinduism. Some young male Hindus even seek castration as a path to religious fulfilment.

Evolutionary psychology suggests that humans and other animals are not driven by pleasure but by the need to survive and to pass on their genes. This would suggest that aggression and sexual promiscuity (in heterosexual males) are the real drivers of human action, not pleasure seeking. If pleasure occurs, it is a by-product not a primary goal. Taken to its logical conclusion the aggressive psychopath represents an evolutionary success.

As an indication of Freud's ambivalence about the role of pleasure, not only did he emphasize the reality principle, he also introduced the competing death instinct into his theory about the human condition. In doing this he emphasized the role of aggression rather than pleasure in normal psychology and so came near to the evolutionist position.

See also: *sadness; creativity; fear; personality disorders; substance misuse.*

FURTHER READING

Freud, S. (1920/1955) 'Beyond the pleasure principle', in the *Collected Works of Sigmund Freud (Volume 18)*. London: Hogarth Press.

Kopp, S. (1973) *If You Meet the Buddha on the Road Kill Him!* New York: Sheldon Press.

Maslow, A.H. (1968) *Toward a Psychology of Being*. Princeton, NJ: Princeton University Press.

Reich, W. (1961) *The Function of the Orgasm*. New York: Farrar, Straus and Giroux.

Rogers, C.R. (1961) *On Becoming a Person*. Boston: Houghton Mifflin.

Seligman, M. and Csikszentmihalyi, M. (2000) 'Positive psychology', *American Psychologist*, 55 (1): 5–14.

Creativity

***Definition:* An act of imagination that leads to a solution to a problem or a novel form of artistic expression.**

Key points: *• The link between mental abnormality and creativity is explored • Psychological and sociological accounts for this link are examined.*

Retrospective analyses of successful historical figures, from different fields, highlight the creative potential that has come to be associated with their distress or madness. This is particularly true of painters, composers and writers but scientists also have high rates of reported psychopathology. Of the many poets and writers cited are Ezra Pound and William Styron, as well as Sylvia Plath and Anne Sexton (both of whom committed suicide). Vincent van Gogh also committed suicide and would probably now be seen as suffering from bi-polar disorder, although he appears in older psychiatric texts as a 'creative psychopath'. This defunct diagnosis (also given to Joan of Arc and T.E. Lawrence) was used in relation to personality disorder.

Many classical composers were noted for their social conformity and for being emotionally unremarkable (e.g. Bach, Mendelssohn, Haydn and Schubert). However, collectively composers have had high rates of mental health problems compared to the general population. Mozart is now thought to have suffered from Gilles de la Tourette's Syndrome (a mixture of nervous tics and obsessive-compulsive symptoms). Handel and Schumann were noted for their dramatic mood swings, with Schumann's work only appearing when he was manic. Schumann was diagnosed retrospectively as suffering from schizophrenia by Eugen Bleuler, the psychiatrist inventing that diagnosis. Some of the best work of Beethoven, including his Ninth and arguably finest symphony, appeared after he became depressed because of his hearing difficulties. Debussy transformed a period of ill health and depression into bursts of creativity. From the Russian romantics, Tchaikovsky and Skryabin were noted for their tortured mental states.

In common parlance today, the term 'artistic temperament' is sometimes a code for 'mentally unstable' and the examples given above suggest that depression can be either an impediment to creativity or its source. A whole musical genre emerged from the depressive state – 'the blues'. The term may be traceable to the skin hue of cold and dejected slaves but it now connotes depression. During the twentieth century, many popular creative artists were described as having a range of psychological problems, including substance misuse, psychosis and suicidal depression, for example Ernest Hemingway, Brendan Behan, Dylan Thomas, Brian Wilson and Nick Drake. The list of famous *performing* artists who have lived recklessly (often abusing substances) and died young is long and includes Judy Garland, Elvis Presley, Janis Joplin, Jimi Hendrix, Brian Jones, Keith Moon, Gram Parsons, Jim Morrison and Kurt Cobain.

It is a moot point whether performers are artists or technicians. However, they are obliged to bring into life an artistic event each time they perform and so, in that basic sense, they are creative. Famous performing artists often have the pressures and pleasures of an erratic lifestyle on the road ('sex, drugs and rock and roll') and the omnipotence and self-indulgence triggered by fame and fortune. Also, the *desire* in performers to be famous might reflect a form of pathological narcissism. Frustration, unhappiness and self-indulgence may accrue, whether or not fame is actually achieved. Descriptions of people with narcissistic and histrionic personality disorder emphasize their unending need for dramatic performance and admiration.

Another field in which the confluence of psychopathology and creativity has been evident is in comedy. Examples here in living memory are Spike Milligan, Tony Hancock and Peter Cook. Humour and wit are good examples of creative reasoning and were the basis of a whole piece of work for Sigmund Freud (*Jokes and Their Relationship to the Unconscious*). Similarly, depth psychologists such as Jung and Winnicott have seen play and playfulness has healing expressions of unconscious life.

Psychological accounts of the co-existence of mental health problems and creativity suggest several factors to consider. Some mental health problems affect the motivational level and focus of the individual involved. People who are manic have unusually high levels of energy, which can be converted into industry. Similarly, conditions in which a-social features predominate allow a person's attention to be sustained in a project. Creative people tend to work very hard at their art or science and can be obsessive, often to the exclusion or detriment of their personal relationships.

Depth psychology would suggest that the unconscious is the source of *both* creativity *and* mental abnormality. Freudians view unconscious impulses as being 'sublimated' into socially acceptable products and that 'regression at the service of the ego' can be observed in some patients. Freud considered the imagination to be neurotic daydreaming. Later psychoanalysts, like Melanie Klein, suggested that creativity represents fixation at infantile stages of development. Fixation at the depressive stage involves a person creatively using their destructive fantasies in a reparative or guilt-ridden way. Fixation at the schizoid phase suggests that the person operates just this side of madness and uses their fantasies to avoid people. This frees or compels them to explore their inner world, intensively and extensively. Klein's emphasis on the role of destructive forces operating in both the imagination and the creative act points up a paradox noted by many.

Thus, an ambivalence exists in depth psychology about whether creative people have ever properly grown up (fixation) or whether they are simply prone to regression. An example of the latter is the Freudian view that painting is a regressed sublimation of the smearing of faeces. The notion that creativity is linked to psychological immaturity is indicated by the study of poets and popular songwriters, who tend to be at their best in adolescence and young adulthood. However, this trend is not evident in other fields.

Some existential therapists, like Rollo May, argue that neurosis is blocked creativity and that to provide therapy to imaginative people might rob them of their achievements. May cites Rilke, who left psychotherapy after discovering its goals: 'if my devils are to leave me, I am afraid my angels will take flight as well'. The emphasis in existentialism is on a state of being, which resists narrow rationality and remains open to all experience. For existential therapists (and some psychoanalysts) the poet John Keats is often quoted favourably by this insight: 'negative capability is when a man is capable of being in uncertainties, mysteries, doubts, without any irritable reaching after fact and reason'. This modern existential view of creativity can be found in older religious traditions of Christian mysticism and Buddhism. For example, St John of the Cross was of the view that 'to come to the knowledge you have not, you must go by a way which you know not'.

A more recent psychological approach to creativity can be found (seemingly oddly) in the study of computers, their use of rules and their ability to be programmed to generate new forms of jazz, symphonic music and drawings. This has been championed by Margaret Boden and is more appealing to those studying cognitive science who eschew the older depth psychology and existentialism.

A social, rather than psychological, framing of creativity suggests other possible accounts. The first, already noted about slavery and 'the blues' is that creativity may be stimulated by collective adversity. Desperate circumstances can ensure that 'necessity is the mother of invention'. The second is to do with consequences rather than causes. Creativity involves transgression – a break with convention. People with mental health problems transgress rules with or without reflection and insight. Creativity can thus be framed as one version of transgression, which happens to find social approval. By contrast, madness is a form of transgression which invites perplexity, pity, fear or ridicule.

The social framing of creativity suggests that it is context dependent and so cannot be described abstractly, as the essential characteristics of individuals. The sources of the acts of transgression might be psychological (as discussed earlier), biological (inherited aptitude) or social (we may learn to be imaginative in the family of school) or some combination.

However, whatever the source, judgements about the *outcome* are always social, as they require others to place a positive or negative value on the creative act.

A good example of the contingent nature of creativity is the reaction to the destruction by fire, in London in May 2004, of many expensive warehoused works of modern art. Some mourned their loss, whereas others thought it comical because they thought the works were trivial and without particular merit. To take a different example, a scientific inventor might produce many prototypes, which are cast aside until one is found which has some practical application. The same industry and imagination went in to all versions but only one found approval, because of its use-value. The willingness to experiment with the absurd (avoiding the trap of Keats's 'fact and reason') means that creative people, like mad people, risk ridicule and social marginalization.

If a fine line might exist between the obsessive crank and the creative genius, depending whether or not others approve of the acts or products, this is also true of religious innovations. Christ wandered in the desert and claimed that he was the son of God. He went berserk in the Temple and ranted and raved. The Buddha abandoned his regal existence and wandered aimlessly in the forest. On observing a sick man, an old man and a corpse he became certain of the possibility of enlightenment about human existence. The Prophet Mohammed felt compelled to retreat into a cave near Mecca, where a command hallucination kept telling him to cry. These religious leaders are now venerated by the majority of the world's population. All of them behaved in a way that would invite a retrospective diagnosis of schizophrenia. They now have excessive credibility, whereas the vast majority of those with a current diagnosis of schizophrenia have little or none.

See also: *stigma; labelling theory; sadness; madness; personality disorders.*

FURTHER READING

Andreasen, N. (1980) 'Mania and creativity', in R.H. Belmaker and H.M. van Praag (eds), *Mania: an Evolving Concept*. New York: Spectrum.

Boden, M. (2004) *The Creative Mind: Myths and Mechanisms*. London: Routledge.

Freud, S. (1905) 'Jokes and their relationship to the unconscious', in the *Standard Edition of the Complete Psychological Works of Sigmund Freud (Volume 8) 1953–1974*. London: Hogarth Press.

Greenacre, P. (1957) 'The childhood of the artist', *Psychoanalytical Studies of the Child*, 12: 47–72.

Jamison, K.R. (1993) *Touched with Fire: Manic Depressive Illness and the Artistic Temperament*. New York: Free Press.

Kubie, L.S. (1958) *Neurotic Distortion of the Creative Process*. Lawrence, KS: University of Kansas Press.
May, R. (1972) *Love and Will*. London: Fontana.
Nettle, D. (2001) *Strong Imagination: Madness, Creativity and Human Nature*. Oxford: Oxford University Press.
Porter, R. (1985) '"The hunger of imagination": approaching Samuel Johnson's melancholy', in W.F. Bynum, R. Porter and M. Shepherd (eds), *The Anatomy of Madness (Volume I)*. London: Tavistock.
Post, F. (1994) 'Creativity and psychopathology: a study of 291 world famous men', *British Journal of Psychiatry*, 165: 22–34.

Lay Views of Mental Health and Illness

***Definition:* Lay views of mental health and illness refer to two sets of descriptions. The first are the accounts of people with mental health problems who speak from their experience. The second are the views from non-patients about the nature of mental health and illness.**

Key points: *• The emergence of a lay perspective on mental health and illness is discussed • Themes from patients' accounts are summarized • Public views of mental health and illness are described.*

The notion of a 'lay' view is traceable to the historical division in Western societies of expert and non-expert knowledge. A binary divide is implied with expertise on one side (seen as superior) and inexpert views on the other (deemed to be inferior). The notions of 'lay preacher' and 'the laity' in Christian churches distinguish clerical authority from its followers or flock. It was extended into secular medical scientific language. For example, when psychoanalysis took hold as a profession, from an early stage a dispute broke out about whether those not qualified in medicine could practice. A liberal view prevailed, supported by Freud, but to this day these practitioners are still called 'lay analysts'.

A full research interest in what non-experts think about mental health and illness is fairly new, probably for two reasons. First, the study of health, whether it is physical or mental, is less easy and appealing to researchers than the study of illness (the patient's experience of disease). Second, without socio-political changes in the role of users of health services, mental health professionals showed very little spontaneous interest in the accounts of 'their' patients. (The latter term, like that of 'follower' or 'flock' implies passivity, with one party forever playing catch up.)

However, these changes did take place. Managers of health and welfare bureaucracies, with political approval and encouragement, increasingly sought the views of service users in order to improve service quality. Moreover, new social health movements critical of professionally dominated models of care began to assert, in very clear terms, their 'lay view'. Below two versions of the latter are summarized, one from patients and the other from non-patients.

- *The patient perspective* Sources of knowledge about the patient perspective come from: user-led surveys (e.g. Read and Baker, 1996); case studies using qualitative methods (e.g. Barham and Hayward, 1991); studies of users' views of mental health services (e.g. Rogers et al., 1993) or specific forms of treatment (e.g. Rose et al., 2004); and demands emerging from the mental health service users' movement (e.g. Chamberlin, 1993). This wide ranging literature points up a number of themes. Patients view their experiences in a variety of ways, with only a minority embracing a model which mirrors a psychiatric diagnosis. Other accounts, based upon social explanations, biographical accounts or spiritual knowledge, are often preferred. These alternative accounts also emphasize the baggage created by a psychiatric diagnosis and patients are often fearful of the negative views this invokes in others. This is well justified as social exclusion is indeed encountered in practice. Complaints from patients are largely about the narrow bio-medical service responses and the personal insensitivity that these create.
- *Lay views of mental health and illness* There are a number of pathways into researching lay views of mental health and illness. The first is to look at legal decision making under the control of juries. Jury verdicts reflect ambivalence about expert knowledge. For example, psychiatric expert witnesses may be believed sometimes but not others. Two famous cases here were of the British mass murderers Peter Sutcliffe and Dennis Nilsen. In these cases, psychiatrists argued

that they suffered from mental disorder (paranoid schizophrenia and psychopathic disorder respectively) but the juries held them to be personally responsible for their actions (Rogers and Pilgrim, 2005). These verdicts seem to reject medical paternalism and may reflect the lack of credibility of psychiatric expertise. In one of the cases (Sutcliffe) interventions from psychiatrists after the trial ensured that he was transferred from prison to a secure hospital, indicating that the lay view did not prevail in the legal process.

A second pathway of understanding is in the study of 'nimby' ('not in my back yard') campaigns (Sayce, 2000). Lay views about people with mental health problems are predictably hostile and distrustful. Stereotypes of mental health problems in antiquity focused on aimless wandering and violence (Rosen, 1968). Studies of stereotypes in modernity show that non-patients still mainly focus on deranged psychotic behaviour and do not mention the commonest of all psychiatric diagnoses: depression (Cochrane, 1983). Moreover, public hostility to psychiatric patients is not merely one of attitude. Read and Baker (1996) asked patients about their encounters with others in the community and nearly half described verbal abuse or physical attacks. Similarly, Campbell and Heginbotham (1991) found hostile action in employers' refusals of candidates who declared previous mental health problems. The stereotypical connection between violence and mental illness was confirmed in large US public surveys (DYG Corporation, 1990; Field Institute, 1984). The vote was split though, indicating that public views are not universally hostile or prejudicial. The problem is that the negative position is sufficiently prevalent to have a discriminatory impact on people with mental health problems.

The third form of understanding of lay views comes from taking personal accounts of mental health (rather than mental illness) (Rogers and Pilgrim, 1997). In the latter study lay people found it extremely difficult to articulate a positive view of mental health and preferred to define it negatively by referring to the avoidance of mental illness. However, they did have views about how to avoid stress and how to positively parent children in order to encourage their well-being. They also believed that the source of mental health problems was mainly related to social stressors but that the solution to problems remained in the hands of the individual sufferer.

See also: *the mental health service users' movement; stigma; social exclusion; risks to and from people with mental health problems; mental health service quality.*

REFERENCES

Barham, P. and Hayward, R. (1991) *From the Mental Patient to the Person*. London: Routledge.

Campbell, T. and Heginbotham, C. (1991) *Mental Illness: Prejudice, Discrimination and the Law.* Aldershot: Dartmouth.

Chamberlin, J. (1993) 'Psychiatric disabilities and the ADA: an advocate's perspective', in L.O. Gostin and H.A. Beyer (eds), *Implementing the Americans with Disability Act.* Baltimore, MD: Brookes.

Cochrane, R. (1983) *The Social Creation of Mental Illness*. London: Longman.

DYG Corporation (1990) *Public Attitudes Toward People with Chronic Mental Illness.* Elmsford, NY: DYG Corporation.

Field Institute (1984) *In Pursuit of Wellness: a Survey of California Adults*. Sacramento, CA: California Department of Mental Health.

Read, J. and Baker, S. (1996) *Not Just Sticks and Stones: a Survey of the Stigma, Taboo and Discrimination Experienced by People with Mental Health Problems*. London: MIND Publications.

Rogers, A. and Pilgrim, D. (1997) 'The contribution of lay knowledge to the understanding and promotion of mental health', *Journal of Mental Health*, 6 (1): 23–35.

Rogers, A. and Pilgrim, D. (2005) *A Sociology of Mental Health and Illness (Third Edition)*. Maidenhead: Open University Press.

Rogers, A., Pilgrim, D. and Lacey, R. (1993) *Experiencing Psychiatry: Users' Views of Services*. Basingstoke: MIND/Macmillan.

Rose, D., Wykes, T., Leese, M., Bindman, J. and Fleischmann, P. (2004) 'Patients' perspective on electro-convulsive therapy: systematic review', *British Medical Journal*, 326: 1363–5.

Rosen, G. (1968) *Madness In Society*. New York: Harper.

Sayce, L. (2000) *From Psychiatric Patient to Citizen: Overcoming Discrimination and Social Exclusion*. Basingstoke: Macmillan.

Eating Disorders

***Definition:* Eating disorders refer to patterns of food consumption which are associated with a detrimental impact upon a person's health and well-being.**

Key points: *• The role of food in the psychological and psychiatric literature is discussed • Features of eating disorders are described and their implications for society explored.*

The relationship between food and mental health appears in the psychological and psychiatric literature in a variety of ways. Three in particular will be mentioned here.

- *Orality and personality* In classical Freudian theory, the oral phase was when the infant experienced pleasure through the mouth during normal psychosexual development. Later, Melanie Klein focussed on the infant's ambivalence towards the breast and accounted for oral passivity and oral aggression in humans in her revision of Freudian theory. These psychoanalytical reflections suggest that a range of oral activities, including greed, food avoidance, food preference and substance misuse, can be accounted for by fixation in the oral phase of life.

  In addition the personal aspects of orality (mood swings, dependency, ambivalence towards others, narcissism and verbal aggression) are also personality characteristics traceable to early infancy, according to psychoanalysts. These adult personality characteristics are deemed to reflect the child's earliest ways of relating, arising first from dependent sucking in the early oral stage and then aggressive biting after the arrival of teeth. Psychoanalysts vary in their views about the significance of the oral stage of development. Some suggest that only the psychoses can be traced to this stage. Others argue that all forms of mental health problem reflect difficulties in early infancy (for a further discussion of the psychoanalytical view of orality, see Rycroft (1969));
- *Obesity* The extent to which obesity can be accounted for by psychological factors is contentious. There are genetic differences in body shape. While weight gain and loss are correlated directly with the amount of calories consumed, genetic loadings amplify or reduce this correlation. Some thin people can eat a lot and gain little weight. In others weight gain occurs readily. A range of health problems (including type II diabetes, cardiovascular disease and some cancers) are linked to obesity, especially extreme obesity. To the extent that obesity is partially linked to exercise levels, there is also a link with mood and anxiety, as the latters are influenced beneficially by exercise. Also weight loss in obese people can be thought of either as a psychological process (emphasizing the central role of the dieter's personal agency) or as a bio-medical problem. In the latter case, the agent of change is not the patient but their treating surgeon, who may intervene with mouth wiring or stomach stapling (for a further discussion of obesity, see Ogden (1996));

- *Eating disorders* Eating disorders (which are described in *DSM* IV and *ICD10*) are only meaningful in cultures in which there is no food scarcity. The tendency to eat excessively and then vomit (bulimia), or to avoid and hide food (anorexia), occurs in cultures in which food is regularly available. Both bulimia and anorexia are more common in females and tend to emerge in adolescence. Bulimia typically emerges in late adolescence but anorexia has an earlier onset. (The incidence of eating disorders is very rare in young children and in older adults.) The typical anorexic girl fears weight gain and considers her body to be too large, even when she is demonstrably underweight. Some patients have alternating phases of binge eating and food avoidance, and may exhibit habits common to both (vomiting and laxative use) throughout. Some other activities, such as excessive exercise also predict anorexia, though the direction of causality is not clear. (Do competitive runners, dancers and gymnasts need to keep their weight down to perform efficiently? Alternatively, are the excessive activity and the eating disorder both parts of a personal strategy to remain thin?)

Eating disorders can occur in isolation but they are often linked to other mental health problems, such as low mood and self-harming. Indeed, both anorexia and bulimia can themselves be framed as self-harming activities, as the patient is denying themselves sustenance to live or they are interfering with their body in an injurious way. Examples of the latter are vomiting, which inflames the oesophagus and rots the teeth and starvation itself which can lead to a range of health problems. The preponderance of eating disorders in girls has led to many feminist accounts (Malson, 1997). These emphasize both social norms (girls aspiring to an 'ideal' model figure) and the control of food and weight as political strategies. The latter may reflect the young girl's access to control, given the relative powerlessness of females in a patriarchal society.

Eating disorders throw into relief a number of features about food and its physical and symbolic relationship to human welfare:

- *Eating disorders indicate a global division between rich and poor* Eating disorders only exist in conditions of dietary plenty for the bulk of the population. While it is true that poor diet and malnutrition are present in the poorest sectors of developed societies, even these may exhibit eating disorders, because food, of sorts, is regularly available. By contrast, in developing countries mass starvation can be common. In these countries the dominant problem is finding something to eat on a regular basis. Eating disorders can only meaningfully arise when the patient has a predictable source of food to regulate – hence they are a product of relative affluence (van Hoecken et al., 1998). For example, studies in Egypt, China and India suggest that anorexia nervosa is not identifiable in their young female populations (Tseng, 2003);

- *Eating behaviour, like all behaviour, is a form of communication* While the precise meaning or range of meanings of eating disorders are open to interpretation and debate, binge eating, food avoidance and a preoccupation with body shape are powerful communications. In particular, the level of risk entailed (in the case of low weight anorexic patients this means a real risk of death) points up the power involved in a person's regulation of their food intake. The religious ritual of fasting emphasizes the trans-historical symbolic significance of this point. Thus eating disorders can be framed as clinical conditions inside individuals but the meaning of a particular patient's behaviour can be framed in its particular communicational context;
- *The gendered nature of eating disorders is indicative of the role of women in society* This point was noted above with the qualifier that men and boys may exhibit eating disorders, albeit less frequently (only around 10% of anorexics are male). The availability of food intake, as a conscious or unconscious psychological strategy to exert personal control in a social context of powerlessness, is central to this gendered picture. Also, the fashion industry has idealized a body shape which is closer to that of young boys than it is of most women, with ready access to food. Moreover, the strong regressive character of female anorexics suggests that life may seem more attractive as a pre-pubescent girl than as a grown up woman. The body shape of the typical adolescent anorexic and the eventual creation of amenorrhea (more than three months without menstruation) support this hypothesis (Bruch, 1974).

Explanations by family therapists that anorexia reflects families which are enmeshed, overprotective, rigid and which fail to resolve conflicts between parents, cannot account for the skewed incidence in girls. (Presumably boys are just as common as girls in such families.) However, they might explain why some girls but not others become anorexic (Minuchin et al., 1978). These explanations may also account for why there is a norm of body consciousness in adolescent girls in Western developed societies, under the pressure of the fashion and dieting industries, but they do not all develop eating disorders;

- *Eating disorders exemplify the problems of mind/body dualism* This point is discussed in relation to physical health in another entry in the book. Not only do psychological factors lead to eating disorders, the latters in turn create physical health problems. Obese people have shorter lives. Those with eating disorders also are at risk of dying young (suicide rates are very high in this group) but in addition they risk physical illnesses from the metabolic disruptions their habits create. Apart from amenorrhea, hair distribution can change and loss of metabolites can create the risk of fitting. Malnutrition may be evident in symptoms such as anaemia, hypoglycaemia (low blood sugar) and osteoporosis (brittle bones). Pubescent anorexics may show growth retardation. For these reasons the treatment or management of eating disorders must involve a biopsychosocial approach from mental health professionals.

See also: *gender; physical health; mental health.*

REFERENCES

Bruch, H. (1974) *Eating Disorders: Anorexia Nervosa and the Person Within*. London: Routledge.

Malson, H.M. (1997) 'Anorexic bodies and the discursive production of feminine excess', in J.M. Ussher (ed.), *Body Talk: the Material and Discursive Regulation of Sexuality, Madness and Reproduction*. London: Routledge.

Minuchin, S., Rosman, B.L. and Baker, L. (1978) *Psychosomatic Families: Anorexia Nervosa in Context*. Cambridge, MA: Harvard University Press.

Ogden, J. (1996) *Health Psychology: a Textbook*. Buckingham: Open University Press.

Rycroft, C. (1969) *A Critical Dictionary of Psychoanalysis*. Harmondsworth: Penguin.

Tseng, W.-S. (2003) *Clinician's Guide to Cultural Psychiatry*. London: Academic Press.

van Hoeken, D., Lucas, A.R. and Hoek, H.W. (1998) 'Epidemiology', in H.W. Hoek, J.L. Treasure and M.A. Katzman (eds), *Neurobiology in the Treatment of Eating Disorders*. Chichester: Wiley.

PART 2

Mental Health Services

Primary Care

Definition: Primary care refers to the first point of contact patients have with a health service. Staffed by general medical practitioners and other health care workers, it provides an initial diagnosis and treatment and it may be the start of a referral pathway to other services.

Key points: • *The importance of primary care for people with mental health problems is discussed* • *Problems associated with the medicalization of psycho-social problems in primary care are outlined.*

Primary care is important for people with mental health problems for three main reasons. First, over 90% of them will be in contact with their general practitioner (GP) or other primary health care worker during a year (Goldberg and Huxley, 1980). Second, only a small minority (around 10%) of such patients are then referred on to specialist mental health services. Consequently, most people with mental health problems only receive a primary care response. Third, in the wake of large hospital closures, most people with a history of psychosis are now living in the community, for most of their lives. Whether or not they return occasionally to acute service inpatient stays, for the most part primary care will be their point of contact with the health service.

There are international differences in the salience of primary care and the above is a summary of the relevance of the current British NHS to people with mental health problems. For example, both the USA and the former Eastern European Communist bloc countries have seen shifts in recent years towards a greater primary care emphasis. Previously in the USA specialist facilities predominated. In the case of the Eastern bloc there were community-based polyclinics.

An implication of a primary *medical* response to mental health problems is that what are essentially psycho-social problems are framed from the outset as medical diagnoses. This is particularly the case with so called 'mild to moderate' mental health problems, which GPs codify as anxiety states and depression. Psychiatric epidemiologists estimate that about 25% of a typical GP case load involves those with a mental health problem, the bulk of which is diagnosed as anxiety or depression (Ustun and Sartorius, 1995). Around a fifth of these patients have persistent symptoms and so consult regularly in primary care (Goldberg et al., 2000). This medical framing is important because it has lead to a predominance of bio-medical interventions (psychotropic drugs). As a result, the drug companies target GPs for psychotropic drug marketing (Lyons, 1996).

This bio-medical emphasis in primary care has led to two credibility problems for this service response. First, the availability of psychological interventions has lagged behind drug treatments (though there are several indications that this is being recognized and changed). Second, social problems are individualized (as medically diagnosed conditions). Moreover, psychiatrists have reinforced this individualizing process by complaining that GPs do not accurately diagnose and that they under-diagnose mental illness (Freeling et al., 1985; Littlejohns et al., 1999). This discourse suggests that psycho-social problems are not medicalized *enough*. Thus, from a psychiatric perspective the problem with primary care is its medical inefficiency. By contrast, critics of medicalization complain of the mystification that a diagnosis of, say, 'depression' brings (Pilgrim and Bentall, 1999).

In the recent British mental health policy context, primary care has been charged with improving services to people with mental health problems in two ways. First, primary care practitioners are now expected to ensure consistent advice and help to people with mental health problems (including patients with a history of psychosis or 'severe mental illness'). Second, all patients should have their mental health needs assessed. Treatment should then be provided directly or by referral to specialist mental health services. The British government at the time of writing also plans an enlargement of the primary care workforce to respond to people with mental health problems. This enlargement includes a thousand psychology graduates to be trained in brief therapy techniques for those with common mental health problems. The intention is also to expand the primary care workforce to include a thousand GPs with a special interest in mental health.

These policy changes directed by the National Framework for Mental Health (DoH, 1999) provide primary care workers with clear aims and objectives, when responding to mental health problems. However, GPs find it much easier to implement other National Service Frameworks, which have harder bio-medical targets to achieve. For example, a study comparing the National Service Framework for coronary heart disease with the one on mental health showed that the former is implemented much more readily than the latter in primary care (Rogers et al., 2002).

Thus, primary care is a site of many contradictions. It deals with psycho-social problems but they are processed and recorded as medical problems. Although mental health problems are diagnosed as illnesses, they are not addressed within a medical framework as convincingly as bodily condition like heart disease. GPs are criticized for their lack of medical knowledge (by psychiatrists) and yet they are responsible for most people with mental health problems. This point now applies to psychotic patients who previously would have lived most of their lives in large institutions. Primary care is the gateway to specialist services but because of limited capacity in the latter, non-specialist staff often are left to manage complex cases.

Primary mental health care is also racialized and gendered. For example, Afro-Caribbean people do not access primary care as often as whites for mental health consultations. Women attend primary care services more than men in general (not just about mental health problems). This pattern alters both the types of intervention offered to those who attend compared to non-attenders. It also skews the population being both diagnosed and referred on to specialist services. More is said about these implications in the sections on Race and Gender.

See also: *acute mental health services; sadness; fear; madness; race; gender.*

REFERENCES

DoH (1999) *A National Service Framework for Mental Health*. London: Stationary Office.

Freeling, P., Rao, B.M., Paykel, E.S., Sireling, L.I. and Burton, R.H. (1985) 'Unrecognized depression in general practice', *British Medical Journal*, 290: 1180–3.

Goldberg, D. and Huxley, P. (1980) *Mental Illness in the Community*. London: Tavistock.

Goldberg, D., Mann, A. and Tylee, A. (2000) 'Psychiatry in primary care', in M.G. Gelder, J.J. Lopez-Ibor and N.C. Andreasen (eds), *The New Oxford Textbook of Psychiatry*. Oxford: Oxford University Press.

Littlejohns, P., Cluzeaut, F., Bale, R., Grimshaw, J., Feder, G. and Moran, S. (1999) 'The quantity and quality of clinical practice guidelines for the management of depression in primary care in the UK', *British Journal of General Practice*, 49: 205–10.

Lyons, M. (1996) 'C .Wright Mills meets Prozac: the relevance of "social emotion" to the sociology of health and illness', in V. James and J. Gabe (eds), *Health and the Sociology of Emotions – Sociology of Health and Illness Monograph*, pp. 55–78.

Pilgrim, D. and Bentall, R.P. (1999) 'The medicalization of misery: a critical realist analysis of the concept of depression', *Journal of Mental Health*, 10 (3): 253–66.

Rogers, A., Campbell, S., Gask, L., Marshall, M., Halliwell, S. and Pickard, S. (2002) 'Some national frameworks are more equal than others: implementing clinical governance for mental health in primary care groups and trusts', *Journal of Mental Health*, 11 (2): 199–212.

Ustun, T.B. and Sartorius, N. (1995) *Mental Illness in General Health Care: an International Study*. Chichester: John Wiley.

Acute Mental Health Services

***Definition:* Acute mental health services are accessed by, or imposed upon, people who are deemed to be in immediate need of containment to assess their needs, or to intervene when they are acting in a very distressed, disturbing or perplexing way.**

Key points: • *The history of acute mental health care is outlined along with its professional advantages to psychiatry* • *Problems on these units are discussed in relation to their social control function* • *Alternatives to inpatient care are considered.*

The 1890 Lunacy Act required that all people entering asylums were detained compulsorily and a certificate of insanity issued. They were 'certified' – a term that is still used in jest in the vernacular today. The 1930 Mental Treatment Act introduced the notion of 'community care' and allowed for 'voluntary boarders'. After the Second World War, the first moves became evident to reduce the size of, or even to abolish, the old large Victorian asylums. However, it was not until the late 1980s that this programme of hospital closures became a reality in most localities.

In the run up to this, during the 1970s, more and more acute psychiatric care was being sited in District General Hospitals. The psychiatric profession advocated this shift in order to raise its status and align itself with other medical specialities, already present in general hospitals (Baruch and Treacher, 1978). The dominance of medical forms of treatment in psychiatry by this period (drugs and electroconvulsive therapy) meant that siting a 'department of psychiatry' in a general hospital was in line with a bio-medical environment of beds, blood tests and drug trolleys. It gave the appearance of scientific medicine coming of age in relation to mental illness.

For a while the co-existence of these new general hospital facilities, alongside the yet-to-be-closed large asylums, meant that the majority of people being admitted to either type of facility were voluntary patients. For example, by the mid-1980s only 8% of admissions were classified as being 'formal' (i.e. involuntary). Even for this period, this figure was probably an under-estimate of the amount of coercion required, as patients reported that they were told to agree to admission as an alternative to compulsion being used. In other words, for as long as the threat of compulsion exists some patients will be under duress to go to hospital voluntarily. These are 'pseudo-voluntary patients' (Rogers, 1993). Indeed, as long as lawful compulsory powers exist to admit patients to a facility then it is impossible to provide an accurate estimate of those who might be genuinely voluntary.

By the time the large Victorian asylums had been closed in the 1990s, the pressure on the small units in general hospitals increased for a number of reasons. First, the availability of beds was dramatically reduced, as the 'backstop' of the asylum acute admission ward disappeared. Second, some (but not all patients) who had been long-term residents in the old hospitals and had moved to community residences, episodically developed crises. Previously these crises had been contained in the long-term hospital. Third, the increasing prevalence of substance misuse, in the poor localities in which many patients with long-term mental health problems had been settled, led to more and more 'dual diagnosis' patients being managed in acute units. Substance misuse increases the chances of chaotic and violent behaviour in psychotic patients.

As a result of these aggregating pressures, the ratio of officially recorded voluntary to involuntary admissions was reversed. By the mid-1990s, the great majority of patients entering acute units did so under a formal section of the civil part of the 1983 Mental Health Act (hence the expression 'sectioned patient'). This altered the prospects for these acute units. In the early 1970s, their advocates in the psychiatric profession aspired to offer medicalized treatment centres for people in acute mental health crises. Thirty years later, at the turn of the century, they had become holding containers for coercively admitted patients who might be intoxicated, chaotic or dangerous. Assaults against staff increased and the units became a site for illicit drug dealing. Risks from patients themselves were joined by others from the local impoverished culture. The function of acute units had been reduced to one of crisis containment. A census of activity in these units in the late 1990s concluded that they were 'non-therapeutic' (Sainsbury Centre for Mental Health, 1998).

However, this scenario had always been likely. The bio-medical ethos and its attendant confidence in the 1970s were never evidence based. They were driven instead by professional rhetoric. The preferred bio-medical reliance on drug treatment brought in its wake adverse effects ('side effects'), which were life diminishing and sometimes were life threatening. Moreover, the titles of these drugs are misleading. 'Anti-psychotic' medication does not cure madness and 'anti-depressants' do not cure sadness (though they alter some symptoms, some of the time, in some people). The psychiatric profession's belief in, and triumphant claim about, a 'pharmacological revolution' has been misplaced. The burgeoning range of drugs produced after the 1950s was not the reason why the large hospitals were closed. The latter occurred for a mixture of financial and ideological reasons. The large hospitals had become too costly for the State and many parties objected to the wholesale segregation of devalued people (Busfield, 1986).

In the past 20 years many critical professionals and disaffected users have pointed out that removing a person from the social context in which their mental health crisis had appeared – and then returning them to the same situation – was not a helpful response. The point was made many years earlier in the classic critique of the mental hospital (Goffman, 1961). Goffman noted that tinkering with problems and using hospitals as a garage for human breakdowns was not a form of service that is likely to be effective. People are not automobiles and so their problems cannot be rectified mechanistically in an isolated setting. Indeed, the notion of 'service' is inherently problematic, if and when compulsion is used – a 'service' to or for whom? Can a 'service' be imposed on a client?

Many involved with acute care are now more than aware of the problems they face, whether or not the above brief analysis of their nature is conceded. A number of points could be made about these challenges. First, staff could accept realistically that the acute services they provide are not likely to create mental health gain in patients, though they might temporarily give some respite to them and their significant others. Second, acute mental health problems might be better understood and managed by offering crisis intervention services in the community, rather than insisting that patients go into hospital. Third, where acute units are being used for purposes of coercive social control (as they are now in the majority of cases) it might be wise to admit to this function and not mystify it with the claim that acute services are simply providing 'treatment under the Mental Health Act'.

See also: *mental health policy; coercion; mental health service quality; substance misuse.*

REFERENCES

Baruch, G. and Treacher, A. (1978) *Psychiatry Observed*. London: Routledge.

Busfield, J. (1986) *Managing Madness*. London: Hutchinson.

Goffman, E. (1961) *Asylums*. Harmondsworth: Penguin.

Rogers, A. (1993) 'Coercion and voluntary admission: an examination of psychiatric patients' views', *Behavioural Sciences and the Law*, 11: 259–67.

Sainsbury Centre for Mental Health (1998) *Acute Problems: a Survey of the Quality of Care in Acute Psychiatric Wards*. London: Sainsbury Centre for Mental Health.

Forensic Mental Health Services

***Definition:* Forensic mental health services detain or treat mentally disordered offenders.**

Key points: *• Secure mental health facilities are described • Problems associated with these facilities are outlined.*

Most of the work of forensic mental health services involves the detention and treatment of offender-patients. In addition, they provide some community support and treatment for mentally disordered offenders released from prisons or discharged from hospital facilities. In Britain, inpatient facilities for mentally disordered offenders are overwhelmingly in the NHS, though some prisons, or units within them, focus on work with those with a diagnosis of personality disorder. Conditions in prison for psychotic patients are extremely poor.

The NHS facilities are layered in security level. There are three high-security hospitals in England (Ashworth, Broadmoor and Rampton) and one in Scotland (Carstairs Hospital). Northern Ireland and Wales have no maximum-security facilities. Smaller medium secure facilities can be found regionally. Many open facilities have locked wards (for example, dealing with dementing patients). These are usually described as 'low secure' environments. Some low secure environments may be rehabilitation services for long-stay offender patients attached to medium secure units.

Under the current Mental Health Act of 1983, mentally disordered offenders are classified in one or more of the following diagnostically related groups: mental illness, psychopathic disorder, mental impairment, severe mental impairment. The latter two groups (with learning disabilities) are mainly detained at Rampton Hospital and smaller regional medium secure units. The physical security levels of these hospitals and units are such that escapes are very rare. The high-security hospitals (until recently called the 'Special Hospital' system) have been controversial in the last 30 years, with official inquiries about care standards and their physical condition being evident in all three. Some of these inquiries have been triggered by 'whistle-blowing staff' and media exposés of mistreatment or corruption. Two of the official inquiry reports in the 1990s (from Blom-Cooper and Fallon) recommended the closure of Special Hospitals.

By and large, the treatment regimes in secure facilities are similar to acute inpatient units for those with a diagnosis of mental illness, combining containment with biological and psychological interventions. However, for those with a diagnosis of personality disorder treatment regimes have been developed which are peculiar to secure settings and in which psychological interventions predominate.

Forensic mental health facilities are permitted to detain patients indefinitely and the average length of stay tends to be at least as long as would be expected had the offender gone to prison for a defined sentence (though this broad correlation contains individual variability). Thus any advantage afforded to offenders going to hospital rather than prison is mainly about the living environment rather than about loss of liberty. Judgements about discharge from secure hospitals are based upon both evidence of improvement in symptoms of mental disorder and reduced risk to others. Because the prediction of re-offending is not perfect, staff making discharge decisions will tend to err in favour of 'false positives', to pre-empt criticism. As a consequence, many patients feel aggrieved that their stay in hospital has been unduly long.

High security mental health facilities are gendered – they are mainly used to contain male offender patients. A small number of female patients are detained at Rampton Hospital system and others dispersed in medium secure facilities. At the same time, prevalence rates of mental disorder in female prisons are higher than in male prisons (but high in both). Male offender patients are much more likely to be sex offenders. Also male offenders are more likely to acquire the label of anti-social personality disorder or psychopathic disorder, whereas women are more likely to be labelled as 'borderline personality disorder'. The offending profile of women is more likely to include infanticide and arson. Substance misuse is prevalent in both groups, as is a history of maltreatment in childhood.

The following controversies have attended secure mental health services:

- *Risk management* This has been double sided. On the one hand, overly liberal risk management can lead to dangerous patients being released who seriously re-offend. On the other hand, the authoritarian culture common in any high-security environment can tilt into negligence and harm to patients (possibly resulting in death). Also, the tendency towards 'false positive' decision making was noted above. Thus a conflict exists in secure environments between efforts to cultivate patient-centred care and third party interests, which ensure the security of others (potential victims in open society). The latter emphasis inevitably encourages a distrustful attitude to detained patients, which can undermine the mutual trust required to create therapeutic optimism;
- *Isolation and institutionalization* Secure facilities have been frequently characterized by professional, organizational and physical isolation. These factors together can lead to what the policy analyst John Martin described as a 'corruption of care' and the mistreatment of patients. At times, organizational isolation can also lead to the risky behaviour of patients going undetected. (For example, at Ashworth Hospital a child was brought in as a visitor to be abused by sex offenders.) Those who have argued for the abolition of the large Special Hospitals have recognized that the varied psychological problems of people in them still require a

response involving containment not just treatment. The issue in this debate has been about size – the larger the number of beds in a residential facility the greater the risk of isolation and institutionalization. While these problems were widespread in 'mental illness' and 'mental handicap' hospitals in the 1960s and 1970s, they rapidly diminished with hospital run down and closure. Because high security hospitals are a remnant of an older network of large institutions, they remain vulnerable to old organizational problems;

- *Problems of indefinite detention* Whatever the mental state of detainees at the outset, indefinite detention brings with it particular forms of demoralization, anger and dysfunctional conduct. This point applies to those in prison as well as in hospital. If an offender faces no prospect of liberty then this affects their mental health. Also, it affects their motivation to collaborate with treatment. They may refuse treatment or they may comply with it disingenuously in order to negotiate their discharge. This poses a particular problem for risk assessors. The risk of offending can be tested ultimately and properly only in open settings. Dealing with long-stay patients is also potentially demoralizing for staff and can make a contribution to the 'corruption of care', noted earlier;
- *The medicalization of criminality* This controversy is mainly in relation to those with a label of anti-social personality disorder or psychopathic disorder. Placing rapists, paedophiles and murderers in a medical setting signals to them that they are not responsible for their actions and this can form a substantial barrier to treatment. (They 'patiently' wait for the medical problem they 'suffer' from to be 'treated'.) All agree that changes in anti-social behaviour rely overwhelmingly on the agency of the offender – they must be responsible for their actions; past, present and future. For this reason, many argue that those with a diagnosis of personality disorder should only be rehabilitated in prisons. This debate has been fuelled further by the question about whether personality disorder is 'treatable' at all. In strict terms it is not (because by definition personality characteristics are stable). However, there is evidence that *offending behaviour* can be altered by psychological interventions even in those with a diagnosis of personality disorder.

Despite the above controversies, a couple of points can be made about secure mental health facilities, which suggest that in some respects they are *less* problematic than those services dealing with nonoffenders. The latter may be detained in acute mental health facilities, without committing an offence. By contrast, offender-patients would warrant detention as prisoners and they would have the protection of due legal process and careful government inspection once detained. Consequently, their detention is consistent with natural justice. By contrast, 'civil' patients (that is those detained under 'civil' sections of the mental health act rather than as 'mentally disordered offenders') are detained without trial. Another point in favour of mentally disordered offenders is that more is spent on them compared to those in contact with open mental health services. However, this financial advantage to mentally disordered offenders applies only to hospital, not prison, placements.

See also: *learning disability; personality disorders; risks to and from people with mental health problems; biological interventions; psychological interventions; acute mental health services.*

FURTHER READING

Blom-Cooper, L. (1992) *Report of the Committee of Inquiry into Complaints about Ashworth Hospital.* London: HMSO.

Gostin, L. (ed.) (1985) *Secure Provision: a Review of Special Services for the Mentally Ill and Mentally Handicapped in England and Wales.* London: Tavistock.

Kaye, C. and Franey, A. (eds) (1998) *Managing High Security Psychiatric Care.* London: Jessica Kingsley Publishers.

McGuire, J. (ed.) (1995) *What Works: Reducing Reoffending.* London: Wiley.

Martin, J.P. (1984) *Hospitals in Trouble.* Oxford: Basil Blackwell.

Monahan, J. and Steadman, H.J. (eds) (1994) *Violence and Mental Disorder.* Chicago: University of Chicago Press.

Van Marle, H. and van den Berg, W. (eds) (1997) *Challenges in Forensic Psychotherapy.* London: Jessica Kingsley Publishers.

Service-user Involvement

***Definition:* User involvement is part of a wider political consensus that those who use public services should have a say in how they are organized and planned. When applied to users of mental health services, it reflects a range of initiatives to include users in: their individual care plans; staff recruitment and training; and service development.**

Key points: *• A brief background to user-involvement policy in Britain is given • Constraints on its development are discussed and estimates of its success are discussed.*

In Britain, mental health service-user involvement is now a well rehearsed and endorsed position from service managers and politicians. With regard to the latter, it reflects both a Thatcherite legacy and a Blairite policy of consumerism in public services. As will be noted again later, it is particularly difficult to reconcile consumerism (with all of its assumptions about voluntary choice) with forms of service provision which have coercion at their centre. The notion of user-as-consumer is only one connotation; Rogers and Pilgrim (2001) note that users also appear in the literature as patients, as survivors and as providers.

This official central government-endorsed consumerist emphasis is important to note because user involvement could be justified in other ways or demanded for other reasons. For example, it could be seen as a human right. Alternatively, it could be used as a Trojan horse by the mental health service users' movement to insinuate oppositional arguments, when disaffected patients are angry with their treatment (in its widest sense), at the hands of services and service professionals.

When user involvement was mooted in the late 1980s, some of those involved in the service users' movement expressed the concern that it might deflect scarce time and energy. This suggested that user involvement was viewed by some more radical users as a form of diversionary co-option (Campbell, 1996; 2001).

Another opening clarification is about relatives of users. In the separate entry on carers, it is noted that sometimes the consumerist position leads to an amalgam discourse from service managers, who will sometimes refer to 'users and carers' in the same phrase. A version of this is 'user and carer involvement'.

As Diamond and colleagues (2003) note, the term 'user involvement' is ambiguous. The most conservative use of the term is in relation to eliciting consumer feedback (Bhui et al., 1998). This is analogous to the consumerist process of, say, hotels asking guests to fill in a satisfaction survey. It involves no direct negotiation between provider and recipient and the former can use their discretion about data utilization. The progressive limits of user involvement are defined by projects which encourage users to be directly involved in service planning or in service improvement (Barnes and Shardlow, 1997; Pilgrim and Waldron, 1998). The conservative aspiration is the easiest to achieve. It is not labour intensive. It requires little or no new financial or workforce resources. It can be acted upon or ignored. It can be cherry picked and selectively attended to. By contrast, the more radical scenario is harder to achieve but if successful its impact on changing services would be greater.

Constraints on the progress of service-user involvement can thus be summarized as follows:

- *The current status of the factors prompting user involvement* It was noted in the introduction that consumerism was the main driver that started user involvement and has been retained. Two other triggering factors were present in the 1980s. The first was the eventual implementation of desegregation (hospital run down and closure). The second was the problem of psychiatric knowledge, which was attacked first by 'anti-psychiatry' and then by the mental health service users' movement.

  These two triggers are still present but their influence may be less than in the past. For example, although the large hospitals were closed, we have also witnessed both trans-institutionalization (the greater presence in prisons of people with mental health problems) and re-institutionalization (the movement of long-stay patients into private hospitals and other smaller residential units). In other words part of the hoped-for success of user involvement was that it would entail partnerships to collaborate on ensuring quality of life in the community. In practice, the community as a central site of user satisfaction is hedged around now by older forms of residential containment. To confirm this more money is currently spent on inpatient facilities than on service changes to make them more community orientated (see section on Financial Aspects). More on the second factor will be noted in the next point;

- *The resilience of the bio-medical approach to care* Since user involvement emerged as a policy in the 1980s, there has been no evidence that a more holistic approach to care has become an established norm in most localities. The balance between biological and psychological interventions remains skewed towards the former for most people in contact with specialist services. While all psychotic patients receive medication (new or old 'anti-psychotics'), only a minority receive psycho-social interventions. This is important because a recurring message from user consultations is that the balance should shift from medication to talking treatments;
- *The lack of money to support user involvement* Central government provides no ring-fenced money to guarantee user involvement. It is left to the discretion of local providers. Pressures on funding in services are such that user involvement could be given a low priority;
- *The ultimate constraint of coercion* As with the retention of bio-medical interventions this is also an important factor. What users recurrently demand is more options and greater voluntarism in their service contact. Pressures on inpatient beds in the last 20 years, since hospital run down, have made acute units into unambiguous sites of coercive social control, with the majority of patients being involuntary and the remaining minority having a questionable voluntary status (Rogers, 1993). Consumerism is based on the assumption that service recipients can take or leave what is offered. Clearly this is not the case with mental health services, where involuntary detention is ever-present. In what sense can the logic of voluntary partnerships, suggested by the notion of user involvement, have any genuine meaning in the context of this coercive service character? Put differently, the more that coercion dominates a service site the less meaning user involvement can have. This may be why those aspects of the service which are voluntary, psychologically orientated and community based tend to receive a stronger endorsement from users (Diamond et al., 2003).

Given these constraints estimates of the success of user involvement have been variable in recent years. Pilgrim and Waldron (1998) reported minor successes in relation to local changes to day centre provision, advocacy services and improved communications with local mental health service professionals. Bowl (1996) in a social service setting found that staff did not manage to successfully share power or build partnership with users and that there were insufficient financial resources to sustain user involvement. Bowl also found staff resistance against involving users in staff selection. (This can be contrasted with many NHS mental health services which now include users on staff selection panels.)

The study of Diamond and colleagues (2003) was more optimistic. They found that success had been achieved in relation to the presence of regular service-user meetings and in user involvement in staff recruitment and in organizing and planning services. There was weaker success reported in relation to involvement in staff training and in contacts with advocacy services. Given these ambiguous results in relation to the early days of user involvement, maybe more time is needed to provide a clear research picture of its success or failure as a policy.

See also: *carers; the mental health service users' movement; mental health policy; segregation; financial aspects of mental health.*

REFERENCES

Barnes, M. and Shardlow, P. (1997) 'From passive recipient to active citizen: participation in mental health user groups', *Journal of Mental Health*, 6: 289–300.

Bhui, K., Aubin, A. and Strathdee, G. (1998) 'Making a reality of user involvement in community mental health services', *Psychiatric Bulletin*, 22: 8–11.

Bowl, R. (1996) 'Involving service users in mental health services: social services departments and the NHS and Community Care Act 1990', *Journal of Mental Health*, 5 (3): 287–303.

Campbell, P. (1996) 'The history of the user movement in the United Kingdom', in T. Heller (ed.), *Mental Health Matters*. Basingstoke: Macmillan.

Campbell, P. (2001) 'Surviving social inclusion', *Clinical Psychology Forum*, 150: 6–13.

Diamond, B., Parkin, G., Morris, K., Bettinis, J. and Bettesworth, C. (2003) 'User involvement: substance or spin?', *Journal of Mental Health*, 12 (6): 613–26.

Pilgrim, D. and Waldron, L. (1998) 'User involvement in mental health services: how far can it go?', *Journal of Mental Health*, 7 (1): 95–104.

Rogers, A. (1993) 'Coercion and voluntary admissions: an examination of psychiatric patients' views', *Behavioural Sciences and the Law*, 11: 259–68.

Rogers, A. and Pilgrim, D. (2001) 'Users and their advocates', in G. Thornicroft and G. Szmukler (eds), *Textbook of Community Psychiatry*. Oxford: Oxford University Press.

Carers

***Definition:* This term is currently used by politicians and health and social care managers to describe the relatives of service users or their significant others.**

Key points: • *Problems with the term 'carer' are described* • *Aspects of the relationships between people with mental health problems and their relatives are outlined.*

It is now common in policy documents about both mental illness and physical disability to see the term 'carers'. It is sometimes used in an amalgam way (as in 'users-and-carers') (Department of Health, 1999; 2002). Both the single and amalgam terms are problematic for a variety of reasons. When people with mental health problems and their significant others are asked, they do not always feel comfortable with the term 'carer'. (Henderson, 2004). The problem is that the convenient social administrative category of 'carer' does not convey accurately the day-to-day complexity of intimate relationships. Dependency in intimate relationships is typically mutual rather than one way, even when one party is sick, impaired or disabled. The highly restricted and one-way connotation of 'carer' and 'cared for' does not do justice to this complexity. Also, the term 'cared for' implies passivity. For this reason, Forbat (2002) has argued that the term 'caree' would be more accurate, as it provides a notion of personal agency on the part of the person who is the identified patient or client.

Given that terms such as 'health care' and 'social care' are administrative descriptions of health and welfare bureaucracies, we also have 'health care' and 'social care' professionals. In the case of those paid to care, the more restricted notion of one-way dependency is more applicable. Generally this is associated with much clearer personal boundaries and role descriptions. The paid carer is not expected to have their personal, social or sexual needs satisfied by those they care for. Indeed, when and if this occurs, then the paid carer is usually deemed to be acting in an unprofessional, unethical or abusive way. By contrast, this moral and legal discourse does not apply to unpaid care. In the latter case, need satisfaction is a two-way process. In the case of paid caring, need satisfaction must be suppressed or managed. It is not merely that one group is paid and the other is not – the way that those cared for or helped or supported is governed by different rules.

With these ambiguities and distinctions in mind, some further points can be made about the notion of 'carer'. Within the broad literature on informal caring in relation to physically disabled people, two features predominate. First, there is a strong feminist critique, which emphasizes that women, more than men, absorb the pressures of unpaid care (e.g. Finch and Groves, 1983). Second, there is an emphasis on 'tending' – the physical support and procedures needed to respond to a physically disabled or sick person.

Neither of these points can be wholly applied in the case of those with mental health problems. In 'mental health care' the need for tending is largely absent in the case of functional problems but extensive in the case of dementia care (see the section on Financial Aspects of Mental Health). Given that living with a person with a diagnosis of functional mental disorder is about coping with a range of tensions in the family, both male and female relatives are drawn into these interpersonal demands and dramas. Thus, when we turn to the peculiarities involved in applying an informal notion of care to mental health, the following points can be made (Rogers and Pilgrim, 2005):

- *Families and aetiology* Some of the professional literature has located intimate family life as the causal source of madness (e.g. Laing and Esterson, 1964). This 'anti-psychiatric' position fell from favour after the 1970s (Howells and Guirgis, 1985). More recently there has been a return to this aetiological theory to an extent (Bentall, 2003);
- *Families and relapse* While the family causation model has been controversial, a consistent professional orthodoxy is that the emotional climate of a family can affect relapse rates in psychotic patients (Jenkins and Karno, 1992; cf. Johnstone,1993);
- *Relatives as risk assessors* The efficiency of risk assessment and prediction (in terms of relapse and risk to self and others) is significantly improved if significant others are included in discussions with staff (Klassen and O'Connor, 1987). However, this can create a role tension for relatives – are they an extension of the mental health system or is their first loyalty to the identified patient? In other words the policy emphasis upon co-opting the views of relatives now

extends to them working on behalf of mental health professionals (Forbat and Henderson, 2003);

- *Relatives as perpetrators and victims of abuse* This links back to the first point about aetiology. Families can be sites of two-way victimization. Relatives of people with mental health problems may sometimes be abusive. Early childhood abuse is a good predictor of a range of mental health problems in adulthood (Briere and Runtz, 1987). In the other direction, the parents of psychiatric patients can be victims of intra-familial violence at times (Estroff and Zimmer, 1994);
- *Relatives as a lobby group* As relatives of those with mental health problems do not work together to advance their own personal liberation, they cannot be described as a full new social movement (see section on Mental Health Service Users' Movement). However, they are an organized mental health policy lobby (Manthorpe, 1984). Organizations such as SANE and Rethink (previously the National Schizophrenia Fellowship) in Britain and the National Alliance for the Mentally Ill in the USA are dominated by relatives of patients. Many of their demands about service improvements are similar to those of the mental health service users' movement. However, they are more likely to prefer a bio-medical model of causation and they place more of an emphasis on the provision of inpatient care and the need for greater coercive control of madness. Despite the tendency to use the amalgam term 'users-and-carers' (noted in the introduction earlier) it is important to note that while both groups have overlapping needs and priorities, these are not identical.

See also: *mental health service users' movement; risks to and from people with mental health problems; financial aspects of mental health.*

REFERENCES

Bentall, R.P. (2003) *Madness Explained: Psychosis and Human Nature*. London: Penguin.

Briere, J. and Runtz, M. (1987) 'Post-sexual abuse trauma: data implications for clinical practice', *Journal of Interpersonal Violence*, 2: 367–79.

Department of Health (1999) *National Service Framework for Mental Health*. London: Department of Health.

Department of Health (2002) *Developing Services for Carers and Families of People with Mental Illness*. London: Department of Health.

Estroff, S. and Zimmer, C. (1994) 'Social networks, social support and violence among persons with severe and persistent mental illness', in J. Monahan and H. Steadman (eds), *Violence and Mental Disorder: Developments in Risk Assessments*. Chicago: Chicago University Press.

Finch, J. and Groves, D. (1983) *A Labour of Love: Women, Work and Caring*. London: Routledge.

Forbat, L. (2002) '"Tinged with bitterness": re-presenting stress in family care', *Disability and Society* ,17 (7): 759–68.

Forbat, L. and Henderson, J. (2003) 'The professionalization of informal carers', in C. Davies (ed.), *The Future of the Health Workforce*. Basingstoke: Palgrave.

Henderson, J. (2004) 'Constructions, meanings and experiences of "care" in mental health'. Unpublished PhD Thesis, Open University, Milton Keynes.

Howells, J.G. and Guirgis, W.R. (1985) *The Family and Schizophrenia*. New York: International Universities Press.

Jenkins, J.H. and Karno, M. (1992) 'The meaning of expressed emotion: theoretical issues raised by cross-national research', *American Journal of Psychiatry*, 149: 9–21.

Johnstone, L. (1993) 'Family management in "schizophrenia": its assumptions and contradictions', *Journal of Mental Health*, 2: 255–69.

Klassen, D. and O'Connor, W. (1987) 'Predicting violence in mental patients: cross-validation of an actuarial scale'. Paper presented at the annual meeting of the American Public Health Association.

Laing, R.D. and Esterson, A. (1964) *Sanity, Madness and the Family*. Harmondsworth: Penguin.

Manthorpe, J. (1984) 'The family and informal care', in N. Malin (ed.), *Implementing Community Care*. Buckingham: Open University Press.

Rogers, A. and Pilgrim, D. (2005) *A Sociology of Mental Health and Illness* (*Third Edition*). Maidenhead: Open University Press.

Mental Health Professionals

***Definition:* The term 'mental health professionals' refers to those who work with people with mental health problems. A variety of occupational groups specialize in the field, notably, psychiatrists, clinical psychologists, mental health nurses, mental health occupational therapists, and mental health social workers. Other groups to be found are counselling psychologists, forensic psychologists, counsellors, psychotherapists and some pharmacists who specialize in mental health work.**

> ***Key points:*** *• The occupational backgrounds of those working with people with mental health problems are outlined • The relationship between these occupational groups is discussed.*

Mental health work is constituted by a range of professionals. The term 'psy complex' is used at times to capture this complexity but is more general, as it also denotes other professional activities informed by psychological approaches (such as teaching and advertising).

Historically, mental health services were politically dominated by the medical specialism of psychiatry, though latterly this dominance is less clear, given the competition evident from other professions. For example, the general management of mental health services is commonly dominated now by mental health nurses. The management of certain client groups (those with a diagnosis of personality disorder or learning disability) is often led by clinical psychologists.

A legal reflection of this shift is the recently proposed English mental health legislation, which replaces the older notion of 'Responsible Medical Officer' with one of 'Clinical Supervisor', which could be held by a 'Consultant Psychologist'. This role is responsible for the admission and discharge of formally detained patients. This highlights the peculiarity of a form of health work, which at times involves coercion and captive clients.

The range of occupational groups mentioned in the definition above is associated with a variety of academic disciplines. Only psychologists have a single academic discipline underpinning their work (psychology). Post-graduate training then transforms and separates this core academic discipline into different applied wings. Clinical psychologists work in a variety of health settings, including but not limited to mental health work, whereas counselling psychologists, a smaller group, mainly do mental health work. Forensic psychologists mainly work in prisons, and less commonly, in health services.

The disciplinary background of the other mental health professions, including medicine, is mixed. For example, medical and nurse training includes inputs from sociology, psychology, pharmacology and neurology. A complication, when discussing the mental health professions, is that the term 'discipline' is used in mental health services to indicate occupational background (as in 'multi-disciplinary team' or 'inter-disciplinary collaboration'). By contrast, in higher education, the term 'discipline' tends to refer to a core body of knowledge (such as mathematics, philosophy, sociology, geology, anatomy, physiology and so on).

As all mental health professionals are now graduates (until quite recently this was not the case for mental health nurses), one way of examining the field of mental health is to explore its diverse knowledge base. The term 'profession' indicates a form of occupation, which is different from a 'worker'. Professionals are defined by the possession of more credentials and their focus on working with people rather than goods. However, in mental health services, at different times, the words 'worker', 'practitioner', 'professional', 'discipline' or 'occupation' can all be used to connote the same notion.

The history of the professions suggests a different bias towards one or other of these meanings. For example, male asylum attendants in the nineteenth century pre-figured psychiatric nursing. They were employed to man-handle and restrain disturbed lunatics. This working class and trade unionized emergent wing of a profession was rejected by mainstream nursing. The latter, under the guidance of Florence Nightingale, was wholly female and middle class. From the outset, these genteel Victorian spinsters saw themselves as professionals not workers. The reverse was the case in what was to become mental health nursing.

The different educational backgrounds of the mental health professionals shape their character. For example, psychiatrists, being trained in medicine, generally work diagnostically and use physical treatments, such as drugs and electroconvulsive therapy. Psychologists, being trained in psychology, are more likely to use formulations about a patient's problems and offer some form of psychological intervention. Nurses vary in between these positions. The lesser professional confidence of mental health nurses is indicated by the continued use of the term 'psychiatric nurse', reflecting the subordinate relationship between medicine and nursing.

These are only general trends of work being described, which typically characterize each occupational group. Exceptions can also be found and are not uncommon. For example, some psychiatrists train as medical psychotherapists and do not prescribe drugs. Some clinical psychologists use diagnostic terms, when assessing patients' problems. Thus approaches to mental health work overlap across the occupational groups.

A consequence of this overlap of roles and approaches across the mental health workforce is that sometimes the identity of a practitioner is defined more by their treatment orientation than by their occupational origins. For example, psychoanalytical psychotherapists from different occupational backgrounds might share a common identity. As a result, an individual practitioner with this orientation may lose their sense of belonging to the occupational group, which originally provided them with the legitimate credentials to do mental health work.

As well as the blurring of roles between groups within mental health work, some mainly trained in the field can be found working outside of specialist mental health services. For example, both clinical psychologists and psychiatrists work with people with physical health problems and those with learning disabilities.

Some forms of treatment for mental health problems imply a traditional division of labour centred on medicine. For example, drug therapy flows from a medical diagnosis and prescribed treatment controlled by psychiatrists. Nurses then are responsible for accurately administering medication on a daily basis (or via less frequent injections) and then monitoring the positive or negative effects of the treatment.

At other times, treatments are controlled autonomously by professionals from different backgrounds, who carry and regulate their own caseloads, with the support of a personally negotiated supervisor. For example, forms of psychological therapy might be deployed autonomously by nurse therapists, psychologists (of different types), medical psychotherapists, social workers or occupational therapists.

Outside of specialist mental health services in the private sector can be found a greater number of counsellors and psychotherapists. The credentials and regulation of these groups is less consistent than in mainstream health service work with people with mental health problems. In order to work in statutory mental health services in Britain, then all professionals must come within the framework of health legislation. They must also demonstrate their competence through specific credentials presented at the point of their appointment and they must demonstrate regular knowledge updates ('continued professional development'). In the private sector, these legal requirements are absent, although to stay registered with a particular parent training body, practitioners must still subscribe to a code of conduct and give a personal commitment to continued professional development.

Finally, the definition of mental health professionals given at the outset focuses on those most closely associated, on a regular basis, with specialist mental health services. However, two other occupational groups are important in regulating access to the latter. First, police officers are involved with mental health crises in the community and their resolution or in securing a specialist referral. Second, GPs are an important gatekeeper into specialist services. They also are involved in the assessment and treatment of the majority of people with 'mild to moderate' mental health problems. GPs are taught that there will be a psychological dimension to around a third of all the patient presentations they see on a daily basis. Therefore, it might be argued that because of the volume of patients they see, GPs are a type of mental health worker.

See also: *psychological interventions; causes and constructs; coercion; learning disability; primary care.*

FURTHER READING

Carpenter, M. (1980) 'Asylum nursing before 1914: a chapter in the history of nursing', in C. Davies (ed.), *Re-writing Nursing History*. London: Croom Helm.
Cheshire, K. and Pilgrim, D. (2004) *A Short Introduction to Clinical Psychology*. London: SAGE Publications.
Gask, L. (2004) *A Short Introduction to Psychiatry*. London: SAGE Publications
Goldie, N. (1978) 'The division of labour amongst mental health professions – a negotiated or an imposed order?', in M. Stacey and M. Reid (eds), *Health and the Division of Labour*. London: Croom Helm.
Saks, M. and Allsop, J. (eds) (2003) *The Regulation of the Health Professions*. London: SAGE Publications.

Biological Interventions

***Definition:* Biological interventions for mental health problems include medication, electro-convulsive therapy (ECT) and psychosurgery.**

Key points: *• Biological interventions are the mainstay of psychiatric treatment though they are sometimes used in combination with psychological interventions • Biological interventions are described and criticisms of them summarized.*

Biological interventions are the mainstay response to mental health problems. These interventions may be offered or imposed alone or in combination with psychological interventions. (Olfson and Pincus, 1999)

The following points summarize biological interventions and the controversies surrounding them:

- *The most prevalent form of intervention is medication* Psychiatric (or psychotropic) drugs are used in the treatment of all forms of mental disorder and there is an evidence base to support their appropriate use (Baldessarini, 1999). For this reason it is virtually unheard of for a person with a mental health problem to be un-medicated. This statement is particularly true for those in contact with specialist mental health service. The psychiatric profession has tended to describe these drugs in relation to their impact on a diagnosed mental disorder (e.g. 'anti-depressants', 'anti-psychotics'). However, before the Second World War this was not the case – drugs were seen only as an adjunct to psychiatric treatment, to suppress or manage symptoms. They were called 'sedatives' or 'tranquillizers'. After the 1950s, the so called 'pharmacological revolution' brought with it a curative rhetoric, encouraged by the pharmaceutical industry (even though the newer drugs still only suppress symptoms);
- *Drugs have been associated with recurrent criticism from their recipients* Because psychotropic drugs, by definition, have powerful effects on the central nervous system, they have been associated with a range of negative or adverse effects. (These are sometimes called 'side effects' which is misleading, as they are not secondary or marginal in the experience of patients.) These effects are often life diminishing and sometimes they can be life threatening (Kellam, 1987; Waddington et al., 1998). As well as individual drugs having effects, which may both reduce symptoms and create problems, the psychiatric profession has been criticized for using cocktails of drugs ('polypharmacy'). Another criticism has been of therapeutic over-dosing ('megadosing'). Both polypharmacy and megadosing have been linked to deaths of recipients (Breggin, 1993). Two high-profile critiques have been associated with the minor and major tranquillizers (Fisher and Greenberg, 1997). The first of these refers to the benzodiazepines, used as anxiolytics (to reduce anxiety symptoms) and hypnotics (to aid sleep). These widely prescribed drugs in primary care were addictive and ineffective after a few weeks. The second group refers to the older anti-psychotic drugs called 'neuroleptics'. These have been associated with three disabling and disfiguring adverse effects: Parkinsonism; tardive dystonias (painful muscle cramps); and tardive dyskinesia (involuntary muscle movements, grimacing, eye rolling and tongue flicking). These problems accumulated over the decades after

the 1950s, as the average prescribed dose level kept rising (Segal et al., 1992);

- *The lack of political concern about some adverse drug effects reflects the low social status of psychiatric patients* In the 1950s when the major tranquillizers were introduced they were used in low doses. As the years progressed and dose levels were raised and cumulative chronic treatment had its effect, more and more patients complained of disabling effects, particularly in relation to tardive dyskinesia. Brown and Funk (1986) note that the 'pandemic' of these drug induced symptoms was only tolerated by society because of the passivity and low social status of chronic psychotic patients. To confirm this, when the National Association for Mental Health (MIND) launched a publicity campaign about the use of major tranquillizers in the 1970s, in conjunction with the popular TV programme *That's Life*, little public concern was forthcoming. However, the programme was overwhelmed by responses about *minor* tranquillizers and the latter became the focus of the campaign thereafter;
- *The use of ECT is less common than medication but it remains a controversial intervention* Although medication dominates the lives of psychiatric patients, ECT is hardly a rare event. In their study of 1000 long-term psychiatric patients, Rogers and colleagues (1993) found that nearly half had received it at some point in their lives. More recent official data suggests that in excess of 11000 patients receive it annually and a fifth of these under conditions of compulsion (Department of Health, 1999). ECT has always been a controversial treatment especially in its early days when patients were shocked without anaesthesia or muscle relaxants (backs were broken from the induced fit). In more recent times the modifications in the procedure have not diminished hostility from its critics (Breggin, 1993). Critics argue that it is frightening to its recipients and that it leads to long-term cognitive deficits (Rose et al., 2003). By contrast, professionals convinced of the treatment's efficacy dismiss user concerns as being unfounded and in the minority (Wheeldon et al., 1999);
- *The use of psychosurgery is rare but highly controversial* This procedure involves cutting or destroying specific parts of the brain in order to treat resistant psychiatric conditions. Its use is now restricted to depressed or obsessive-compulsive patients who are unaffected by all other forms of intervention. Its use diminished after the 1950s when there was clear cumulative evidence of permanent adverse effects including apathy, epilepsy and intellectual impairment. The ethical

concerns about the procedure are threefold: first, by their nature randomized controlled trials cannot be conducted and evidence has to rely on case follow up; second, the intervention is irreversible; third, adverse effects can be very serious (Merskey, 1999).

A final point to make about biological treatments is that their prevalence is driven by the preference by the psychiatric profession for somatic solutions to psychological problems and by the support of the pharmaceutical industry for research into the use of medication.

See also: *psychological interventions; the mental health services users' movement; 'anti-psychiatry'; the pharmaceutical industry.*

REFERENCES

Baldessarini, R.J. (1999) 'Psychopharmacology', in A.M. Nicholi (ed.), *The Harvard Guide to Psychiatry*. London: Harvard University Press.

Breggin, P. (1993) *Toxic Psychiatry*. London: Fontana.

Brown, P. and Funk, S.C. (1986) 'Tardive dyskinesia: barriers to the professional recognition of iatrogenic disease', *Journal of Health and Social Behaviour*, 27: 116–32.

Department of Health (1999) 'Electroconvulsive therapy: survey covering the period January1999 to March 1999', *Statistical Bulletin 22*. London: Department of Health.

Fisher, S. and Greenberg, R.P. (eds) (1997) *From Placebo to Panacea: Putting Psychiatric Drugs to the Test*. New York: Wiley.

Kellam, A.M.P. (1987) 'The neuroleptic syndrome so called: a review of the literature', *British Journal of Psychiatry*, 150: 752–9.

Merskey, H. (1999) 'Ethical aspects of physical manipulation of the brain', in S. Bloch, P. Chodoff and S.A. Green (eds), *Ethical Aspects of Drug Treatment*. Oxford: Oxford University Press.

Olfson, M. and Pincus, H.A. (1999) 'Outpatient psychotherapy in the United States: the National Medical Expenditure Survey', in N.E. Miller and K.M. Magruder (eds), *Cost Effectiveness of Psychotherapy*. New York: Oxford University Press.

Rogers, A., Pilgrim, D. and Lacey, R. (1993) *Experiencing Psychiatry: Users' Views of Services*. Basingstoke: MIND/Macmillan.

Rose, D., Wykes, T., Leese, M., Bindman, J. and Fleischmann, P. (2003) 'Patients' perspective on electro-convulsive therapy: systematic review', *British Medical Journal*, 326: 1363–5.

Segal, S.P., Cohen, D. and Marder, S.P. (1992) 'Neuroleptic medication and prescription practices with sheltered care residents – a 12 year perspective', *American Journal of Public Health*, 82 (6): 846–52.

Waddington, J.L., Yuseff, H.A and Kinsella, A. (1998) 'Mortality in schizophrenia. Antipsychotic polypharmacy and absence of adjunctive anticholinergics over the course of a 10-year prospective study', *British Journal of Psychiatry*, 173 (10): 325–9.

Wheeldon, T.J., Robertson, C., Eagles, J.M. and Reid, I. (1999) 'The views and outcomes of consenting and non-consenting patients receiving ECT', *Psychological Medicine*, 29: 221–3.

Psychological Interventions

***Definition:* The use of conversations or other inter-personal methods to ameliorate mental health problems.**

Key points: *• Psychological interventions are outlined • The problematic link between psychological theory and these interventions is discussed • Questions of effectiveness of psychological interventions are raised.*

Psychological interventions are referred to variously in the professional mental health literature as, 'psychological therapies', 'talking treatments', 'psychotherapy' or 'counselling'. They are characterized by forms of stylized conversations with patients (or 'clients'), intended to create mental health gain. There is an explicit taboo on physical contact. This provides an immediate appeal to patients, as they are seemingly less interventionist than biological treatments. There are some exceptions though. For example, there are some 'body therapies' which involve physical contact. Also, some methods are barely conversational. An example of this would be the use of impersonally delivered positive reinforcement or aversive stimuli in the use of some behavioural techniques. By and large though, the great bulk of what are described as 'psychological interventions' involve systematized conversations.

When psychological interventions are deployed by professionals, they negotiate therapeutic contracts with clients and deploy explicit rationales for their work. These rationales are wide and varied and reflect the lack of consensus, within both the culture of mental health professionals and of academic psychologists, about how to understand the relationship between experience and behaviour (Cheshire and Pilgrim, 2004). In very broad terms, the types of psychological approach, which underpin interventions, can be identified as: psychoanalysis, behaviourism, cognitivism, humanism, existentialism, general systems theory and postmodernism. Reviews of the relationship of these theoretical trends to clinical interventions can be found in Dryden (2002).

The link between psychological theory and therapeutic practice is far from straightforward. Some interventions are hybrids, which contain elements of several underpinning theories. The very commonly deployed 'cognitive-behavioural therapy' (or 'cognitive-behaviour therapy', 'CBT' or just 'cognitive therapy') contains a particular contradiction. It is an elaboration of behaviour therapy, which can be traced to the application of behaviourism – a form of psychology which deems inner events to be difficult or impossible to study scientifically. By contrast, cognitivism (or cognitive science) privileges the study of inner events. Moreover, the link with cognitivism in contemporary academic psychology is tenuous. The original champions of cognitive therapy were not applied by cognitive psychologists but psychiatrists, who were developing pragmatic alternatives to psychoanalytical therapy (Beck, 1976; Ellis, 1994). This emphasis on the pragmatics of therapy being privileged over theory can also be found in solution-focused brief therapy, a derivative of family therapy (Hawkes et al., 1998).

Psychological interventions may be used by mental health professionals with natural groups (family therapy), stranger groups (group therapy) or with individuals. Also therapeutic communities are whole system treatment regimes, which contain a mixture of small and large groups (with or without some individual work). The therapeutic community approach evolved in residential settings and can be traced to the 'moral treatment' of the early asylum system run by lay administrators, before medical superintendents ushered in their preferred physical approaches. The main spur to the therapeutic community movement during the twentieth century was the challenge of treating a large number of 'shell shocked' combatants but latterly the focus has been mainly on those with a diagnosis of personality disorder or substance misuse (Kennard, 1998).

The cost-effectiveness of conversational methods of treatment has been debated at length with different reviewers offering a range of views. At the critical end of this spectrum, some argue that psychological therapies are dangerous and should be avoided by prospective clients (Masson, 1988). At the other end are those who argue that properly conducted therapy provides demonstrable benefits in response to most mental health problems (Dobson and Craig, 1998). The latter conclusion is about the evidence base supporting therapists who demonstrate 'treatment fidelity' or 'treatment integrity'. That is, they consistently conduct themselves in accordance with the rationale of a specified therapeutic approach.

The gap between the two positions of appraisal may be accounted for by the fact that *in practice* there are always some therapists who are either incompetent or abusive – they lack treatment integrity or they are exploitative. These therapists are actively harmful and provoke what the literature describes as 'deterioration effects'. This group of therapists is important to identify in services because in psychological interventions, the relationship is the main instrument of change and the benign and supportive features of the therapist predict good outcome (Lambert and Bergin, 1983). They are also important for the overall credibility of talking treatments, because they make the difference between positive and negative aggregate outcomes. The very reputation of psychological therapies depends on competent, non-abusive practitioners.

Pilgrim (1997) noted the evidence to support the following complex picture about psychological interventions:

- The overall evidence is that benign supportive conversations are helpful to people. What is less clear is whether any particular professional *rationale* for helpful conversations is superior to another;
- The evidence about treatment integrity suggests that professionals are more effective if they are consistently self-disciplined when applying a rationale for their work. However, lay people with no training can use conversations in an effective way to create psychological improvement in others (they may not *want the helping role* though);
- While there are few demonstrable differences in outcome *between* different theoretical approaches, there are wide variations in outcome achieved by therapists *within* any particular therapeutic approach. This suggests that the *quality* of a relationship is more important than the psychological theory preferred to *understand* it (reinforcing the first point above);
- There are no strong differences in the outcomes achieved by new and very experienced therapists. Again this suggests that helpful interpersonal processes may not be linked to the sophistication of the helper but to some other factor;
- People change for the better when not in therapy. This suggests that other variables (including lay relationships) create mental health gain. What is called 'spontaneous remission' may be misleading because it implies that psychological processes are not operating outside of a professional arena – it may understate the power of informal mutual support. If this is the case, then those benefiting most from service contact are probably those whose natural networks are sparse or lacking in supportive relationships.

Despite the ambiguity surrounding the safety and mode of effectiveness of talking treatments, they are frequently a preferred alternative to biological interventions – the mainstay response offered to people with mental health problems. Underlying this grateful endorsement is the shared acculturated idea in modern Western societies that good relationships re-build or enhance mental health. For this reason, psychological interventions, unlike biological ones, are 'anxiously sought and gratefully received'.

Some postmodern critics have noted that therapy inscribes an identity onto its clients in voluntary relationships, derived from its own discourse of what it is to be properly human. For example Rose (1996) talks of the freedom offered by therapy being 'enacted only at the price of relying on experts of the soul'. Similarly, de Swaan (1991) also talks of clients being 'protoprofessionalized' by a therapy culture – learning the world view of a therapeutic ideology in advance of ever becoming a client. In other words, therapists do not simply respond neutrally to problems in living but they also seek to shape the way life should be led. Nonetheless, de Swaan concludes that, 'granted all that is wrong with the helping professions . . . most Europeans and Americans may still be suffering more from a lack of what these have to offer than from an overdose'.

See also: *biological interventions; the mental health services users' movement.*

REFERENCES

Beck, A.T. (1976) *Cognitive Therapy and the Emotional Disorders*. New York: Meridian.

Cheshire, K. and Pilgrim, D. (2004) *A Short Introduction to Clinical Psychology*. London: SAGE Publications.

de Swaan, A. (1991) *The Management of Normality*. London: Routledge.

Dobson, K.S. and Craig, K.D. (eds) (1998) *Empirically Supported Therapies: Best Practice in Professional Psychology*. London: SAGE Publications.

Dryden, W. (ed.) (2002) *Handbook of Individual Therapy*. London: SAGE Publications.

Ellis, A. (1994) *Reason and Emotion in Psychotherapy: Revised and Updated*. New York: Birch Lane Press.

Hawkes, D., Marsh, T. and Wigosh, R. (1998) *Solution-focused Therapy: a Handbook for Healthcare Professionals*. Oxford: Butterworth/Heinemann.

Kennard, D. (1998) *An Introduction to Therapeutic Communities*. London: Jessica Kingsley.

Lambert, M.J. and Bergin, A.E. (1983) 'Therapist characteristics and their contribution to psychotherapy outcome', in C.E. Walker (ed.), *The Handbook of Clinical Psychology Vol. I*. Homewood: Dow Jones-Irwin.

Masson, J. (1988) *Against Therapy*. London: HarperCollins.

Pilgrim, D. (1997) *Psychotherapy and Society*. London: SAGE Publications.

Rose, N. (1996) *Inventing Ourselves*. Cambridge: Cambridge University Press.

Financial Aspects of Mental Health

***Definition:* Mental health has health economic implications in two senses. First, the amount of money spent on mental health services can be calculated. Second, the economic consequences of mental health problems can be estimated.**

Key points: • *The amount of money spent on mental health services and the economic consequences of mental health problems will be considered.*

SPENDING ON MENTAL HEALTH SERVICES

In the British context, this has been summarized most recently by the Sainsbury Centre for Mental Health report (2003). Although government spending was increased after 2000, in order to expand the volume of mental health services available, the report concludes that, in practice, this intention is unlikely to be successful. A number of factors support this conclusion. First, although mental health is designated as a priority in health care policy, proportionally the growth in expenditure on it, compared to other areas in local government and the NHS, has been slower. As a result, in proportional terms, the share allocated by the local State to mental health services in now actually falling.

A second indicator of mental health falling behind is the slow progress in the timetable to implement the National Service Framework for Mental Health (Department of Health, 1999). The Sainsbury report estimates that in order to meet the deadlines, current expenditure allocated by central government for mental health services would need to be doubled.

A third factor, indicating that mental health services continue to have a 'Cinderella' status, relates to the range of peculiar costs or budgetary pressures experienced by them. These include debt repayment, staff shortages (which lead to expensive short-term agency payments) and the increasing prescribing costs, associated with the introduction of new and expensive psychotropic medications. A look at the breakdown of spending on mental health services reveals socio-political priorities (see Table 1).

Table 1 *Expenditure by service category in 2002–3*

	Per cent
Community mental health teams	17.2
Access and crisis services	6.6
Clinical services including acute inpatient care	24.6
Secure and high dependency provision	12.3
Continuing care	12.2
Services for mentally disordered offenders	1.1
Other community and hospital professional teams/specialists	1.6
Psychological therapy services	4.6
Home support services	2.1
Day services	5.3
Support services	1.5
Services for carers	0.3
Accommodation	10.3
Mental health promotion	0.1
Direct payments	0.1
Total direct costs	100.0

Source: Sainsbury Centre for Mental Health, 2003

The salience of any item or combined items will vary from reader to reader, according to their value framework. Here one reading will be given. First, there is a socio-political emphasis on social control. Look at the combined items on acute facilities, secure provision and mentally disordered offenders. Between them they account for nearly 40% of government spending on mental health services. This can be compared with the amount spent on mental health promotion – a mere 0.1%. Second, psychological therapy services only receive 4.6% of spending (suggesting a bio-medical inertia in the mental health care system). Third, other non-hospital-based services, which are meant to signal a service re-configuration towards community based interventions are lagging behind the political rhetoric of the chapter on mental health in the NHS Plan (Department of Health, 2000). Between them the items on new assertive outreach, crisis resolution, early intervention and services for carers, account for less than 7% of spending.

THE COST OF MENTAL HEALTH PROBLEMS

A range of studies in Europe and North America have estimated the economic cost of mental health problems. A caution when reading these is that they start from and reinforce a discourse of burden. For example, they do not include estimates of positive contributions arising from the role of creativity in society (see the section on Creativity) or on the role of user involvement, user-led services or the supportive or caring role some of those with mental health problems can provide to their families (Szmukler, 1996). Nonetheless, the burden discourse has legitimacy in a context in which social order and economic efficiency dominate socio-political priorities.

Knapp (2001) discusses economic burden under several headings, which will be summarized here:

- Labour market features are important. Only 20% of psychotic patients are in paid employment (Foster et al., 1996). About a third of sickness absence from work is attributable to 'minor' mental health problems (Jenkins, 1985). The direction of causality is contested about labour market disadvantage (Rogers and Pilgrim, 2003) (see section on Social Class). For psychotic conditions, employer discrimination is clear (Campbell and Heginbotham, 1991). For anxiety states and depression it is more likely that the primary disability of the symptoms means that patients are unable to work. Knapp (2001) summarizes three main points under this heading. First, patients not working become socially excluded (like other unemployed people). Second, the welfare payments to them are a toll on the tax payer. Third, where near full employment is the case in the economy, sickness absence due to mental health problems leads to productivity losses;
- Some studies emphasize economic family impact. For example, relatives may need to transport patients to and from mental health facilities or outpatient appointments (Creed et al., 1997) and may be out of pocket in their ancillary role to State provision (Schene et al., 1996). Families which contain psychotic patients are estimated to spend around 6 to 9 hours per day in ways which limit their social activity or which are experienced as stressful (Magliano et al., 1998). In the case of senile dementia, relatives can be involved for up to 45 hours per week in unpaid care (Cavallo and Fattore, 1997);

- Premature death is also noteworthy. For people with a diagnosis of schizophrenia the risk of death is 1.6 times greater (controlled for age and gender) than the general population. Premature death rates in all diagnostic groups are higher than in the general population (Harris and Barraclough, 1998) but especially for those who abuse substances or who have an eating disorder. Much, but not all, of this mortality profile occurs because of raised rates of suicide. Premature death of those of working age removes them from both the labour market and from welfare burden, if they were unemployed. As Knapp (2001) notes, these brutal economic gains and marginal losses to productivity have to be set against the personal and social loss involved;
- Mentally disordered offenders, although small, constitute a group which creates multiple costs. There are the direct costs to victims and their insurers. Those to the criminal justice system have to be included as well. It should be emphasized, though, that both of these are also applicable to non-mentally disordered offenders. Over and above these, patient offenders have some unique costs, attached to their assessment and 'disposal' into forensic mental health services. These are much more costly per capita than prison facilities;
- Welfare payments to people with mental health problems in the mid-1990s in Britain came to more than £7 billion (Patel and Knapp, 1998). People with mild to moderate mental health problems are a specific burden on sickness and invalidity benefits, prompting the British government recently to offer new rehabilitation services for them to work – the 'Pathways to Work' scheme.

A final point to note is that the political discourse about burden often focuses on 'severe and enduring mental illness' – largely a code for those diagnosed with schizophrenia. However, only 10% of the global burden is accounted for by this group – more than half is accounted for by anxiety and depression (Andrews and Henderson, 2000). This highlights how policy decisions about 'burden' may sometimes be skewed by considerations other than equity of service allocation based on diagnostic prevalence, such as the need to exercise social control over madness in general, and dangerous madness in particular. This reinforces the need to analyse tables, like the one cited earlier, with a political, as well as a financial, eye.

See also: *creativity; social exclusion; social class; suicide; madness; sadness; fear.*

REFERENCES

Andrews, G. and Henderson, S. (eds) (2000) *Unmet Need in Psychiatry*. Cambridge: Cambridge University Press.

Campbell, T. and Heginbotham, C. (1991) *Mental Illness: Prejudice, Discrimination and the Law*. Aldershot: Dartmouth.

Cavallo, M.C. and Fattore, G. (1997) 'The economic and social burden of Alzheimer's Disease on families in the Lombardy region', *Alzheimer's Disease and Associated Disorders*, 11 (4): 184–90.

Creed, F., Mbaya, P., Lancashire, S., Tomenson, B., Williams, B. and Holme, S. (1997) 'Cost effectiveness of day and inpatient psychiatric treatment. Results of a randomised controlled trial', *British Medical Journal*, 314: 1381–5.

Department of Health (1999) *National Framework for Mental Health*. London: HMSO.

Department of Health (2000) *The NHS Plan*. London: HMSO.

Foster, K., Meltzer, H., Gill, B. and Hinds, K. (1996) *Adults with Psychotic Disorder Living in the Community. OPCS Survey of Psychiatric Morbidity*. London: HMSO.

Harris, E.C. and Barraclough, B. (1998) 'Excess mortality of mental disorder', *British Journal of Psychiatry*, 173: 11–53.

Jenkins, R. (1985) 'Minor psychiatric disorder in employed young men and women and its contribution to sickness absence', *British Journal of Industrial Medicine*, 42: 147–53.

Knapp, M. (2001) 'The costs of mental disorder', in G. Thornicroft and G. Szmukler (eds), *Textbook of Community Psychiatry*. Oxford: Oxford University Press.

Magliano, L., Fadden, G., Madianos, M., Caldas de Almeida, J.M., Held, T., Guarneri, M., Marasco, C., Tosini, P. and Maj, M. (1998) 'Burden on the families of patients with schizophrenia', *Social Psychiatry and Psychiatric Epidemiology*, 33: 405–12.

Patel, A. and Knapp, M.R.J. (1998) 'Cost of mental illness in England', *Mental Illness Review Research*, 5: 4–10.

Rogers, A. and Pilgrim, D. (2003) *Mental Health and Inequality*. Basingstoke: Palgrave.

Sainsbury Centre for Mental Health (2003) *Money for Mental Health: a Review of Public Spending on Mental Health Care*. London: Sainsbury Centre for Mental Health.

Schene, A.H., Tessler, R.C. and Gamache, G.M. (1996) 'Caregiving in severe mental illness. Conceptualization and measurement', in H.C. Knudsen and G. Thornicroft (eds), *Mental Health Service Evaluation*. Cambridge: Cambridge University Press.

Szmukler, G. (1996) 'From family "burden" to caregiving', *Psychiatric Bulletin*, 20: 449–51.

Mental Health Service Quality

Definition: The quality of a mental health service can be judged by several criteria including: the amount of mental health gain produced; the proven cost-effectiveness of specific interventions deployed; and improved quality of life for the recipient. In addition, secure mental health services might be judged by their success in containing their residents.

Key points: • *Mental health service quality can be defined by several criteria* • *These implicate the interests of professionals, service users and a range of third parties* • *Given the contradictions involved in the notion of 'service quality', an ethical framework of best practice is implied.*

A more elaborate version of this entry can be found in Pilgrim (1997). In the latter, three main questions were posed:

1 Are professional interventions effective?
2 Are professional interventions acceptable to their recipients?
3 What enhances the quality of life of people with mental health problems?

In answering these questions, a number of contradictions and uncertainties about service quality emerge.

- *The effectiveness of interventions* The majority of the interventions (biological and psychological) used in mental health services have an evidence base for their effectiveness. However, some interventions remain un-researched (particularly when treating complex problems) and there is an imperfect understanding about the effect of multiple concurrent interventions. That is, mental health services often contain a range of interventions but we do not fully understand the way in which they interact. There may be synergies. Alternatively, different approaches may confuse patients and impacts may counteract one another. At other times, where there is research evidence for synergies (as in the concurrent use of biological and psychological interventions, with those with a diagnosis of depression or schizophrenia) this may not be put into regular practice in services (Fadden, 1997).

Also, the use of randomized controlled trials (RCTs) to test the effectiveness of a treatment may lead to misleading conclusions. For example, Brugha and Lindsay (1996) point out that RCTs 'are conducted in unrepresentative ways on unrepresentative and willing subjects. Should it be surprising that, perhaps, the same "good outcomes" might not occur in clinical practice?'. A further problem is that a treatment may be effective at controlling symptoms but generate adverse effects to the detriment of the patient's quality of life. In these circumstances the patient may refuse treatment or accept it resentfully. This can highlight a tension between treatment effectiveness, as defined by the patient, and that defined by third parties, such as professionals and relatives (Finn et al., 1990);

- *Acceptability to recipients* Mental health service contact brings with it certain risks to users. Both can generate adverse effects, although biological treatments are complained about more than psychological ones. The very fact that a new social movement has emerged, which talks of 'surviving' mental health service contact, suggests that users do not find service contact acceptable, much of the time. In part this reflects the coercive role of services and the amount of surveillance users are subjected to during community living. There are other areas of medicine where effectiveness is no better than in psychiatry. This suggests that acceptability (and, in this case, complaints about it) is a function of the patient's total experience of service contact, rather than a measure of effectiveness. A treatment may be effective but not acceptable – again this may be the case in other areas of medicine. However, mental health services seem to demonstrate this contradiction more than others. Another contradiction is that loss of liberty *ipso facto* is unacceptable to detained patients but their inability to abscond might be a positive criterion of service quality used in secure services.

The centrality of service-user confidence in services, as a defining feature of service quality, has been highlighted in the Department of Health's document *Standards for Better Health* (2004), which starts with the statement: 'everyone who comes into contact with the NHS deserves to feel confident in the standard of care they receive'. However, in mental health services the notion of 'standard of care' is not simply defined by patients. In addition, responses to the needs of third parties are embedded in their daily operations. This is the main reason why psychiatric patients often do not 'feel confident in the standard of care they receive';

- *Improved quality of life* Some argue that the ultimate test of service quality is its impact on the quality of life of people with mental health problems living in the community (Brugha and Lindsay, 1996). With de-institutionalization, judgements about service quality increasingly expanded the definition from effective interventions, to include the obligation of services to respond to the social needs of patients (Falloon and Fadden, 1993; Huxley, 1990). As far as secure services are concerned, if patients lose their liberty for long periods of time, then the quality of their life *within* the residential setting can become the main criterion of service quality.

Given the contradictions about service quality generated by these points, then an ethical framework to guide best practice for professionals and mental health managers and policy makers is implied. One such framework is offered by Seedhouse (1993). He suggests that the following five criteria should be applied to maximize service quality:

1 *Openness and humility from professionals*: given the uncertainties about quality and the different ways in which different parties might define it, professionals should be open about their dilemmas. They need to be transparent about what they do and do not know in their work, as well as about the contradictions implied by working for more than one party. They need to offer genuine informed choice about treatments – and when choice is not being offered be honest about this;
2 *Standard setting*: this has two aspects. First, the rhetoric of evidence-based practice should be put into practice. Protocols about treatment integrity (the proper and consistent use of a type of treatment supported by evidence) should be used in services. Second, the definition of desirable treatment outcomes should attend to their acceptability to service users. They should not be limited to professional definitions of effectiveness;
3 *Managerial clarity about purpose*: with the exception of the management of community services, in which only genuine voluntary

relationships are present, all residential facilities (be they acute or forensic services) entail coercive social control. This point cannot be evaded by managers or, if it is, the purpose of mental health services will be mystified. A clear and comprehensive clarification of the purpose(s) of mental health services constitutes this third ethical stricture about service quality;

4 *Professionals' willingness to specify what they do*: as well as being open in general (first stricture above), professionals should also be clear to service users about what they do and why they are doing it. This fourth stricture follows from all three others above;
5 *Genuine partnerships with service users*: user involvement in mental health services is now a commonplace policy. This final stricture implies that the implementation of the policy should be maximized.

See also: *psychological interventions; biological interventions; forensic mental health services; the mental health service users' movement.*

REFERENCES

Brugha, T.S. and Lindsay, F. (1996) 'Quality of mental health service care: the forgotten pathway from process to outcome', *Social Psychiatry and Psychiatric Epidemiology*, 31: 89–98.

Department of Health (2004) *Standards for Better Health*. London: Department of Health.

Fadden, G. (1997) 'Implementation of family interventions in routine clinical practice following staff training programs: a major cause for concern', *Journal of Mental Health*, 6 (6): 599–612.

Falloon, I. and Fadden, G. (1993) *Integrated Mental Health Care*. Cambridge: Cambridge University Press.

Finn, S.E., Bailey, M., Schultz, R.T. and Faber, R. (1990) 'Subjective utility ratings of neuroleptics in treating schizophrenia', *Psychological Medicine*, 20: 843–8.

Huxley, P. (1990) *Effective Community Mental Health Services*. Aldershot: Avebury.

Pilgrim, D. (1997) 'Some reflections on "quality" and "mental health"', *Journal of Mental Health*, 6 (6): 567–76.

Seedhouse, D. (1993) *Fortress NHS: a Philosophical Review of the National Health Service*. London: Wiley.

PART 3

Mental Health and Society

– Mental Health Policy –

Definition: This refers to any society's attempts to promote mental health and to ameliorate mental health problems. It includes legislative arrangements and politically prescribed forms of professional duty and service response.

Key points: • *Mental health policy changes over time in the developed countries of the world are summarized* • *Some differences between these policy trends and policy events in the lesser developed countries are discussed.*

The notion of mental health policy is relatively recent. Until the twentieth century there was a lunacy policy, which gave way gradually to a mental illness policy. It was noted in the first section (Mental Health) that the use of the term 'mental health', as a prefix to 'policy', 'problems' or 'services', is a recent euphemism. However, it is our current discourse and so this entry will use the term as if it is not problematic.

What this initial disclaimer does do, though, is help us to unpick layers of relevant policies which have accumulated over time. Also, this story over time is not fixed and universal. Most of the research on mental health policy has been about mapping changes over time in Western Europe, North America and Australasia. In the developing countries much of this historical pattern is inapplicable. For this reason the dominant picture in the developed countries will be summarized and then some counter-examples given from other parts of the world.

SUMMARY OF SHIFTS IN MENTAL HEALTH POLICY IN THE DEVELOPED COUNTRIES

Western Europe contains the old colonial powers and so has the longest history to summarize. The export of European cultures to the Americas and Australasia after the Middle Ages, means that not all of the following applies to them. In the sixteenth and seventeenth centuries in Europe, the insane either wandered free or they were constrained or cared for in religious dwellings. Madness at this point was not seen as a medical but a social and supernatural problem.

The next change was the loose development of many small private madhouses in the eighteenth century. A few famous large madhouses, like Bedlam in London (opened in 1408), the Casa de Orates in Valencia (1408) and the Hopital General in Paris (1656), predated this period. Although Michel Foucault (1965) in his *Madness and Civilization* dates the 'Great Confinement' of madness in Europe to the Paris institution, in England a full State system of lunatic asylums did not emerge until the nineteenth century (Goodwin, 1997; Rogers and Pilgrim, 2002).

The First World War brought neurosis within the ambit of psychiatry and enlarged its activities to community-based interventions. However, between the First and Second World War (and after the latter) it was still hospital-based psychiatry, with its preference for biological interventions, which predominated. What the twentieth century then saw was two cultures of patients being treated – one in the community (with access sometime to psychological interventions) and another which was still warehoused for long periods in large old asylums and treated wholly with physical interventions. The latter represented the persistent bio-medical position of hospital-based psychiatry, dating from the mid-nineteenth century and still existing today.

During the twentieth century, the psychiatric jurisdiction over psychotic and neurotic patients was enlarged further, as those with personality problems and addictions were added. This is why now we see this admixture of diagnoses in mental health services. Running alongside these changes in professional jurisdiction were formal adjustments to mental health legislation, which defined professional powers of detention and intervention and stipulated safeguards both for patients and against the unfair detention of the sane. In Britain these legislative changes occurred in 1930, 1959 and 1983. Another revision of mental health law is imminent at the time of writing. In the past 50 years, a final and more nebulous layer of mental health policy has been in relation to mental health promotion (see the section with this title).

Hospital run down in Western Europe occurred rapidly in the 1980s (see section on Segregation), with community care being both the great hope of radical reformers and a focus of anger and derision from paternalistic interest groups seeking a return to greater institutional control of mental disorder. The phase of post-hospital closure we currently inhabit is characterized by three key policy processes:

- First, there is the tendency towards re-institutionalization. This refers to the tendency to return to the days of smaller private madhouses (albeit now including, and built outwards from, the State funded acute units);
- Second, there is now evidence of trans-institutionalization. This refers to the evidence that some patients who previously would have been contained in the Victorian asylums now spend long periods of time in jail. Another area of policy debate is in relation to the adequacy of housing, employment and other aspects of social inclusion, for community-based patients (see section on Social Exclusion);
- A third policy challenge for those still committed to social inclusion is in relation to public education about the range and nature of mental health problems. Negative stereotypes are currently being maintained by hostile and deriding coverage of mental health problems in the mass media (see section on this topic).

MENTAL HEALTH POLICY IN DEVELOPING COUNTRIES

The colonial impact of European states was reflected in mental health policy in a particular way. On the one hand Western (especially Germanic) views about insanity were exported. On the other hand, the mass segregation of the pauper insane by the State was absent. For example in India there was an immediate but weak mirroring of the English asylum concept. However, the provision was overwhelmingly for *white* patients. There were regional differences in the administration of these lunatic asylums and they were financially driven. Also the class composition of imperial power meant that the Indian asylum system had to make unusual provision to respond to the social status of British rulers who became insane (Ernst, 1985). While European asylums overwhelmingly dealt with pauper lunatics, on colonized soil abroad the mad were more likely to be from a much higher social class. By the end of the nineteenth century the scale of 'European asylums abroad' declined radically, as the colonial power steadily withdrew its presence.

Most developing countries have had much less hospital-based psychiatry. In some it was simply absent during the twentieth century (e.g. Laos (Westermeyer and Kroll, 1978)). In others it arrived very late (e.g. not until 1961 in Nepal) (Nepal, 2001). By the time asylum beds were peaking in Europe in the mid-twentieth century, the Indian sub-continent had few hospitals or mental health workers. For example, by 1947 England had 15 times more psychiatric beds than India with only 10% of its population (Murthy, 2001).

A paradoxical advantage of this lack of resources for mental health care development in the developing world is that there was less of an institutional infra-structure to remove or displace, when community models of care came into favour (German, 1975; Wig, 1999). A community-based or primary care-driven mental health policy was a socio-economic necessity, created by a scarcity of resources. Because madness was segregated with less frequency, recovery rates for those with a diagnosis of schizophrenia have been higher in developing countries than in Western Europe and the USA (Warner, 1985).

In the light of the discrepancies in resources for mental health policies between the developed and developing countries, the World Health Organization (2000) has suggested a global policy with three prongs. First, there should be more resources allocated to mental health care in all countries, but especially in the developing ones. Second, resource re-distribution is needed *within* health care systems to benefit mental health services (the latter is relatively under-funded in developed countries, compared to physical health care). Third, programmes of collaborative shared care should be developed between State-funded mental health services and voluntary bodies, religious bodies, families, community organizations and patients.

See also: *segregation; mental health; coercion; mental health promotion.*

REFERENCES

Ernst, W. (1985) 'Asylums in alien places: the treatment of the European insane in British India', in W.F. Bynum, R. Porter and M. Shepherd (eds), *The Anatomy of Madness (Volume III)*. London: Tavistock.

Foucault, M. (1965) *Madness and Civilization*. New York: Random House.

German, A. (1975) 'Trends in psychiatry in Black Africa', in S. Arieti and G. Chrzanowski (eds), *New Dimensions in Psychiatry: a World View*. New York: Wiley.

Goodwin, S. (1997) *Comparative Mental Health Policy*. London: SAGE Publications.

Murthy, R.S. (ed.) (2001) *Mental Health in India 1950–2000*. Bangalore: People's Action for Mental Health.

Nepal, M.K. (2001) 'Mental health in Nepal', in R.S. Murthy (ed.), *Mental Health in India 1950–2000*. Bangalore: People's Action for Mental Health.

Rogers, A. and Pilgrim, D. (2002) *Mental Health Policy in Britain*. Basingstoke: Palgrave.

Warner, R. (1985) *Recovery from Schizophrenia: Psychiatry and Political Economy*. London: Routledge.

Westermeyer, J. and Kroll, J. (1978) 'Violence and mental illness in a peasant society: characteristics of violent behaviours and folk use of restraints', *British Journal of Psychiatry*, 133: 529–41.

Wig, N.N. (1999) 'Development of regional and national mental health programmes', in G. de Girolamo (ed.), *Promoting Mental Health Internationally*. London: Royal College of Psychiatrists.

World Health Organization (2000) *World Health Report, Health Systems: Improving Performance*. Geneva: World Health Organization.

Mental Health Promotion

Definition: Like mental health, mental health promotion has been defined in a variety of ways. Common or recurring strands include the promotion of: happiness, the right to freedom and productivity, the absence of mental illness, and the fulfilment of an individual's emotional, intellectual and spiritual potential.

Key points: • *The relationship between mental health promotion and the primary prevention of mental illness is considered* • *The range of factors which are implicated in both of these closely related concepts is outlined.*

The promotion of psychological well-being is closely linked to the primary prevention of mental health problems. The subtle distinction is that in the former case, positive mental health has to be defined, as one or more desired outcomes. In the latter case there needs to be a demonstration that the probability of diagnosed mental illness is reduced. A danger of conflating mental health promotion with the primary prevention of mental illness is that it may maintain a medical focus on a limited clinical population and not address the population's needs as a whole (Tudor, 1996).

The World Health Organization (1986) has offered a view of mental health promotion – the ability of individuals to 'have the basic opportunity to develop and use their health potential to live socially and economically productive lives'. In 1986 the Organization launched a campaign to implement a charter for action to achieve health for all by 2000 and beyond. Later, the Organization emphasized that 'the concept of health potential encompasses both physical and mental health and must be viewed in the context of personal development throughout the life span' (World Health Organization, 1991).

The primary prevention of mental illness can be distinguished from secondary and tertiary prevention. Secondary prevention refers to nipping mental health problems 'in the bud' following early detection. Tertiary prevention refers to lowering the probability of relapse in those with chronic mental health problems.

The distinction but also the relationship between promotion and primary prevention was also made clear by Albee (1993), who used two versions of an equation using similar factors (see Figure 2).

Figure 2 *Preventing mental illness and promoting mental health*

1 Incidence of mental illness = $\dfrac{\text{stress + exploitation + organic factors}}{\text{support + self-esteem building + coping skills}}$

2 Promotion of mental health = $\dfrac{\text{coping skills + environment + self esteem}}{\text{stress + exploitation + organic factors}}$

The factors in the two equations can be addressed one by one:

- *Stress* In the entry on social class it is noted that stress accounts for some of the differences in diagnosis between poorer and richer people. While both groups have adverse and positive experiences, the ratio between the two is different, with the richer group having more buffering positive experiences. Those exposed to lower levels of personal and environmental stress are more likely to be mentally healthy. Conversely, the higher the level of stress, be it acute and severe (trauma) or chronic and low level, the higher the probability of a person developing a mental health problem;
- *Exploitation* The exploitation of individuals, whether it is financial or related to physical, sexual or emotional abuse, increases the risk of mental health problems. Conversely, a person not exposed to these versions of exploitation is more likely to maintain their mental health. The discourse of exploitation is not common in the psychiatric and psychological literature (Sartorius and Henderson, 1992). This may

reflect the tendency of the two disciplines to avoid the language of politics, which might bring accusations of unscientific bias and risk undermining professional credibility. However, a problem for the human sciences is that they are intrinsically about human relationships. Exploitation and other expressions of power differentials are part of the landscape, in some form or other, at all levels of all human societies. Another reason that professionals do not typically address the question of exploitation is that it is beyond their immediate control. The scope of their interventions is limited to the micro-level. This refers to the coping strategies of individuals (Persaud, 1997), family interventions (Dwivedi, 1997) and, at its most extensive, local community psychology initiatives (Rappaport et al., 1984). By contrast, political factors, which manifestly affect the possibility of developing mental health for all, in line with the World Health Organization's expectation noted earlier, are out of the direct and privileged control of professionals. These include measures to prevent starvation and warfare and to ensure that all citizens are well housed and educated and protected from the prejudicial actions of others (Sartorius, 2001);

- *Organic factors* These refer to environmental toxins and stressors and to biological susceptibility. The entries on causes and concept and on social class discuss the latter. The former refers to poisons (such as lead and petrochemicals) which damage the nervous system. They also refer to behavioural stressors, which are then mediated by physiological mechanisms to produce brain damage. The most common example of this is in relation to raised blood pressure increasing the risk of stroke and dementia. The stressors here include insecure work conditions, noisy and dangerous living environments and lifestyle habits such as quality of diet and exercise levels;
- *Social support* This is a crucial buffer against mental health problems. Chronic personal isolation increases the risk of both depression and psychosis. Both are reduced in probability in those people who are part of a supportive social network of primary group (be it close friends or family);
- *Self-esteem building* This refers to early family life and its capacity for developing confidence in the growing child. It also refers to the presence of benign and affirming current relationships – linking back to points above about exploitation and social support;
- *Coping skills* The ingenuity in coping with adversity varies from person to person and probably links back to personal styles learned in the family and at school. Much of the work of cognitive therapists is

devoted to enabling patients lacking these coping skills normally to learn new ones. Conversely, those studying positive psychology have identified those of us who excel at being positive across a range of social contexts.

These factors demonstrate that positive mental health and the primary prevention of mental illness implicate a wide range of factors, which are political, social, psychological and biological. Strategically, mental health promotion requires changes in both public policies (N.B. plural) and public education (Tones and Tilford, 1994). For example, a number of apparently separate policies can affect mental health related to, among others: environmental pollution, child protection, employment, leisure, street cleaning, traffic levels, parenting, schooling, diet and exercise.

The approach taken to mental health promotion and primary prevention reflects the constructs used by those intervening (be they politicians or health and welfare professionals). The list of public policy implications for mental health, noted in the list above, reflect a *social* model of mental health. Those who emphasize psychological determinism would limit their interest to individual and family life. Those who emphasize bio-determinism would emphasize biological interventions (such as genetic counselling and early intervention for psychosis). At its most extreme, this might culminate in a eugenic policy to prevent mental illness.

See also: *mental health; eugenics; causes and constructs; coercion; biological interventions; psychological interventions; physical health; warfare.*

REFERENCES

Albee, G. (1993) 'The fourth revolution', in D. Trent and C. Reed (eds), *Promotion of Mental Health (Volume III)*. London: Avebury.

Dwivedi, K.N. (ed.) (1997) *Enhancing Parenting Skills*. Chichester: John Wiley.

Persaud, R. (1997) *Staying Sane: How to Make Your Mind Work for You*. London: Metro.

Rappaport, C., Swift, C. and Hess, R. (eds) (1984) *Studies in Empowerment: Steps Towards Understanding and Action*. New York: Haworth Press.

Sartorius, N. (2001) 'Primary prevention of mental disorders', in G. Thornicroft and G. Szmuckler (eds), *Textbook of Community Psychiatry*. Oxford: Oxford University Press.

Sartorius, N. and Henderson, A.S. (1992) 'The neglect of prevention in psychiatry', *Australian and New Zealand Journal of Psychiatry*, 26: 550–3.

Tones, K. and Tilford, S. (1994) *Health Education: Effectiveness, Efficiency and Equity*. London: Chapman Hall.

Tudor, K. (1996) *Mental Health Promotion: Paradigms and Practice*. London: Routledge.

World Health Organization (1986) *Health Promotion: Concepts and Principles in Action*. Copenhagen: WHO European Regional Office.

World Health Organization (1991) *Implications for the Field of Mental Health of the European Targets for Attaining Health for All.* Copenhagen: WHO European Regional Office.

Segregation

***Definition:* The imposed separation of one social group from another or from the general population. The term sometimes refers to the isolation of one person.**

Key points: *• The history of the segregation of madness is outlined • Competing ideas about segregation and desegregation policies are discussed • The trans-historical trend of the public rejection of madness is noted.*

The mass segregation of pauper lunatics took place over the final three centuries of the second millennium in Europe and North America. Psychiatric historians do not agree on the precise timing of this societal shift or on the exact explanation for its occurrence (Grob, 1973; Foucault, 1965; Rothman, 1971; Scull, 1979). Some argue that the segregation of lunacy reflected a moral shift in an industrial age of increasing rationality and efficiency (which, of its nature, madness defies). Others argued that class interests in capitalist societies dictated the need to split off and control an economically burdensome underclass (the 'lumpenproletariat'). The destitute, old, sick and infirm were taken into workhouses. The mad and foolish were eventually accommodated in the asylum system during the nineteenth century. Prior to that, they could be found in workhouses and in private or charitable madhouses.

The volume of segregated madness peaked during the 1950s in most countries. It then steadily declined, with a sharp drop off after 1980. The latter marked the eventual implementation of 'desegregation', which has also been called 'decarceration', 'de-institutionalization' and 'community care'. In Britain, the term 'community care' was first mentioned in the

1930 Mental Treatment Act but it only developed common currency in the 1980s. The explanations for desegregation have also been varied (Busfield, 1986; Goodwin, 1997; Rogers and Pilgrim, 2005; Scull, 1983). These competing (or sometimes additive) explanations have included: the introduction of new psychiatric drugs; the fiscal crisis created for the welfare state of costly large institutions; and a shift in professional concerns about appropriate treatment and its setting.

A tension that has been inherent to both the segregation and desegregation policy trends relates to the possibility of social re-integration. That is, therapeutic pessimists have argued for the need to manage chronicity. The therapeutic optimists have argued for the cure or rehabilitation of madness. The pessimists were content to permanently warehouse madness from society, with lunatics permanently living and then dying in the asylum. The optimists hoped to reverse madness and to permit liberty. Examples of the latter in the nineteenth century included the moral treatment used by religious non-medical administrators of asylums (such as, the Quaker Retreat at York) and the early efforts at physical treatment offered by the medical superintendents, who formed the early profession of psychiatry after the mid-nineteenth century (Digby, 1985).

Despite hopes of lunacy policy reformers, the moral treatment of the older charitable asylums, like the Retreat, failed to transfer to the State-run asylum system and custodialism prevailed (Donnelly, 1983). Moreover, although moral treatment ostensibly was more humane, it still was a form of social control and even used physical restraint at times (Castel, 1985; Tomes, 1985). Similarly, during the twentieth century, there were therapeutic optimists championing both biological and psychological interventions. At the same time, others have argued that the quality of life of chronic patients and the need for genuine asylum, not cure, should be policy priorities.

Moreover, the shift from custodialism to professional therapeutic optimism in the second half of the twentieth century was not always appreciated by patients (especially ECT, insulin-coma-therapy and psycho-surgery). Other innovations, such as industrial therapy, were less offensive but were often menial and arguably exploitative. The old segregated asylums had advantages though (compared to the poor urban environments occupied by many chronic patients today). They were typically in large semi-rural spacious grounds with an estate often including a farm, which occupied some patients and provided produce for the hospital. Also, the internal living areas were more spacious than the cramped, low-ceiling environment of many acute mental health units today.

An indication that madness, once segregated, was deemed to reflect a form of lesser humanity was the concern expressed in society, at the turn of the twentieth century, about unfair detention. This showed the willingness of society to split off one group, which could be incarcerated and assaulted with impunity (the insane) from another, whose personal sensitivities and right to autonomy, privacy and physical safety should be fully respected (the sane). Most of the concerns about segregation, thereafter, have not been about the *existence* of segregation but about its proper application. Since the 1920s, reforms of mental health legislation have resonated with this point, as they spell out the circumstances and safeguards required for the imposition of legitimate rather than unfair psychiatric detention.

Another manifestation of this 'two groups of humanity' mentality was the concern expressed after the 1970s about the 'political abuse of psychiatry' (Bloch and Reddaway, 1977). Reports of psychiatrists using enforced psychiatric diagnosis and life-diminishing treatments (major tranquillizers) on political dissidents created an international scandal. However, an implication of the outrage it produced was that enforced psychiatric treatments, which were life diminishing, were legitimate impositions on those who were truly mentally ill. The lack of outrage about the latter indicates that the general public are still prone to accept that the insane do not warrant the rights of full humanity.

Another example about the mass mentality of the sane, faced with madness in its midst, is given by Jodelet (1991). In a social experiment since 1900, at Ainay-le-Chateau in France, patients have been fostered by families in the community. However, they are still separated psychologically by their hosts, who fear contagion and violence and who do not permit sexual relationships between patients and non-patients. On the rare occasion that sexual relationships have developed, the couple has been banished from the community.

A final historical continuity to mention under this entry is individual segregation. In the eighteenth century chains were used to restrain mad individuals. By the end of the nineteenth century padded cells and straight-jackets were used. By the end of the twentieth century unpadded strip cells or seclusion rooms had come into fashion in secure hospitals and acute mental health settings. This remains the case today, although 'seclusion' (in prison the same process is called 'solitary confinement') is seen as a problematic practice and so its minimal use is preferred by mental health professionals. Even today there are parts of the former Communist Eastern bloc (the Czech Republic, Slovenia and Slovakia) where cages are found in large psychiatric institutions. Seclusion rooms and cages indicate that physical segregation is still very much part of the current institutional landscape of psychiatry.

Current mental health services, in developed societies, still fulfil a function of segregation. However, their bed capacity is much more restricted. Acute mental health services only have a fraction of the beds of the old large institutions and they are charged with moving people on as soon as possible. By contrast, the old large hospitals were places of permanent residence and by the end of their days they were often called 'long stay' institutions. The forensic system, of high and medium secure mental health services, offers this residual long-stay function of the Victorian asylum system but is not on the same scale as the old network of asylums.

The reduction in the number of beds in the State sector of mental health services has been compensated for, to some extent, by the development of private facilities to segregate those with mental health problems whose disruptiveness or economic burden cannot be dealt with in community settings. This can be thought of as 're-segregation' or 're-institutionalization' and may mark a return to a form of residential policy similar to the eighteenth century (Pilgrim and Rogers, 1996). Also, rates of mental disorder in prison populations have increased, suggesting that a deviant group once in the asylum system may be now be detained elsewhere. A second re-adjustment made about the function of segregation, the closure of the majority of the large hospitals, has been legal. Mental health legislation has been adapted to include forms of surveillance and options for rapid re-hospitalization for patients now living in the community. Services now are a mixture of small acute units, assertive outreach, outpatient clinics, home treatment services and day centres. At the time of writing the proposed new Mental Health Act for England and Wales reflects this re-adjustment, as it focuses on the control of patients in a range of settings other than in hospital (the emphasis of prior mental health legislation in 1983, 1959, 1930 and 1890).

See also: *risks to and from people with mental health problems; biological interventions; mental health; mental health policy; madness; forensic mental health services.*

REFERENCES

Bloch, S. and Reddaway, M. (1977) *Psychiatric Terror: How Soviet Psychiatry is Used to Suppress Dissent*. New York: Basic Books.

Busfield, J. (1986) *Managing Madness*. London: Hutchinson.

Castel, R. (1985) 'Moral treatment: mental therapy and social control in the nineteenth century', in S. Cohen and A. Scull (eds), *Social Control and the State*. Oxford: Basil

Blackwell.
Digby, A. (1985) 'Moral treatment at the retreat 1796–1846', in W.F. Bynum, R. Porter and M. Shepherd (eds), *The Anatomy of Madness. Vol. II*. London: Tavistock.
Donnelly, M. (1983) *Managing the Mind*. London: Tavistock.
Foucault, M. (1965) *Madness and Civilization*. New York: Random House.
Goodwin, S. (1997) *Comparative Mental Health Policy: from Institutional to Community Care*. London: SAGE Publications.
Grob, G. (1973) *Mental Institutions in America: Social Policy to 1875*. New York: Free Press.
Jodelet, D. (1991) *Madness and Social Representations*. London: Harvester Wheatsheaf.
Pilgrim, D. and Rogers, A. (1996) 'Something old, something new . . . sociology and the organization of psychiatry', *Sociology*, 28 (2): 521–38.
Rogers, A., and Pilgrim, D. (2005) *A Sociology of Mental Health and Illness (Third Edition)*. Maidenhead: Open University Press.
Rothman, D. (1971) *The Discovery of the Asylum: Social Order and Disorder in the New Republic*. Boston: Little Brown.
Scull, A. (1979) *Museums of Madness: the Social Organization of Insanity in Nineteenth Century England*. London: Allen Lane.
Scull, A. (1983) *Decarceration*. Oxford: Polity.
Tomes, N. (1985) 'The great restraint controversy: a comparative perspective on Anglo-American psychiatry in the nineteenth century', in W.F. Bynum, R. Porter and M. Shepherd (eds), *The Anatomy of Madness. Vol. III*. London: Tavistock.

Coercion

***Definition:* The use of, or threat of, force in order to ensure a human being complies with the wishes of others. In the context of mental health services coercion ensures compulsory detention, compulsory treatment or compulsory isolation.**

Key points: *• The circumstances under which psychiatric coercion occurs are described • A continuum of engagement between voluntarism and coercion is discussed • Ethical challenges to psychiatric coercion are highlighted.*

One of the most controversial aspects of mental health services is their association with coercion. At the centre of this controversy is the ethical norm that adult human beings do not coerce others. The typical lawful exception to this is when people break the criminal law. Under these circumstances the police are given delegated lawful powers of coercive detention. What makes mental health services unique is that equivalent powers are lawfully delegated to health workers to control mental disorder and that liberty may be deprived without trial, even when no crime has been committed.

Broadly, there are three circumstances when this happens. First, mentally disordered offenders may be compulsorily detained in forensic mental health services. Second (and more frequently) people with mental health problems, who have not committed a criminal offence, are detained or treated against their wishes. At the time of writing, in Britain, the conditions under which these groups are coerced are described under the 1983 Mental Health Act, with sections of the Act, which refer to 'mentally disordered offenders', being separated from those about 'civil' patients. Third, in some countries there are legal powers to provide involuntary treatment in community settings.

The probability of coercion is predicted, to some extent, by diagnosis. Those with diagnoses of functional psychosis or anti-social personality disorder are treated more coercively – the former in acute mental health services and the latter in forensic mental health services. The other group of patients subject to raised levels of coercion are those who are profoundly depressed and actively suicidal.

Szmuckler and Appelbaum (2001) point out that coercion is the most extreme point on a continuum of engagement between mental health professionals and patients. At the other end of the continuum is completely voluntary contact, initiated and maintained by the client. Some commentators such as deSwaan (1991) have noted that even this point involves patients being acculturated to expect and demand treatment from professionals ('protoprofessionalization') raising a question about the nature of voluntarism.

Further towards coercion, from pure voluntarism, are four gradations of influence, on what Szmuckler and Appelbaum describe as a 'spectrum of pressures':

- *Persuasion*: a patient may be reasoned with and reminded of the consequences of not co-operating with treatment in the past;
- *Leverage*: here a professional might express disappointment in the client's non-co-operative stance. This might lead to co-operation if the client is dependent on the professional;
- *Inducements*: the patient may be offered advantages related to

community living in exchange for treatment compliance;
- *Threat*: here the patient is told that, regretfully, if they do not agree to treatment or hospitalization, then formal powers of compulsion will be invoked; they are made an offer they cannot refuse.

This spectrum or continuum between voluntary and involuntary personal engagement exists in a formal legal context in developed countries. Libertarian critics of mental health law point out that as long as the threat of involuntary detention and treatment exists, then the point of genuine voluntary contact on the continuum becomes meaningless (Szasz, 1970). Certainly, patient accounts of officially entering hospital informally or voluntarily suggest that the common use of threat of coercion leads to many being recorded as being voluntary but they are really 'pseudo-voluntary' patients (Rogers, 1993). This also raises a more general point about conceptualizing the spectrum noted above – it has subjective as well as objective indicators. For example, a voluntary patient may *feel* coerced even when there is no formal record of coercion being evident and coercion is denied by the treating professionals (Hiday, 1992).

Coercion is thought to be warranted, by professionals and others, on two broad grounds. First, there is the paternalistic justification that psychiatric patients often do not recognize the need for treatment, therefore others have to act in their interests to protect their health and well-being. Second, sometimes there is a need to protect third parties. (Together these two points are also captured in the phrase 'risk to self or others'.)

Ethical questions arise on both fronts about discrimination against people with mental health problems. In relation to the preventative paternalistic motive, there are many examples of those without mental health problems, who act in a self-injurious way and where enforced medical paternalism could play an effective preventative role. Common examples are cigarette smoking and excessive eating. However, smokers and obese people are not detained without trial or treated compulsorily. With regard to danger to others, speeding driving and drunken violence can lead to detention (even here not inevitably). However, when this occurs it is after due legal process has been applied and only in relation to past proven action not *potential* action, on the part of the perpetrator. Thus, although ethical grounds can be invoked to justify psychiatric coercion, these grounds can be substantially challenged. It is also clear that the ways in which rules of coercion are differentially applied to people with mental health problems, means that they suffer discrimination.

Coercion has played a role in discussions of both secondary and tertiary prevention of mental illness. Secondary prevention involves nipping an illness in the bud, when early symptoms appear. Tertiary prevention is about staving off relapse in those already ill. An example of the latter is the professional eagerness to ensure compliance with medication in psychotic patients, in order to prevent relapse and the need for hospitalization. With regard to secondary prevention, there has been a recent controversy about early intervention in psychosis. Those in favour of this would like to have powers to ensure treatment compliance in those seen to be at risk. Those against this aspiration point out that prediction of actual psychosis in individuals is difficult and it places those who would not go on to become psychotic at risk of the adverse effects of medication (Bentall and Morrison, 2002; cf. Miller and McGlashan, 2003).

For the foreseeable future, it is likely that in developed societies legal powers will be maintained and occasionally reformed in order to ensure that people with mental health problems are removed from society and are obliged to accept treatment. It is also likely that substantial ethical controversy and some political opposition will continue to surround both of these trends. Aside from the question of human rights violations, when coercion is applied by one human being on another, mental health professionals also struggle with the knowledge that the more that they are seen to coerce, the less likely it is that patients will contact them for help voluntarily. The known presence of recurrent coercion in mental health services encourages people with mental health problems to evade contact.

See also: *risks to and from people with mental health problems; segregation; mental health policy.*

REFERENCES

Bentall, R.P. and Morrison, A.P. (2002) 'More harm than good: the case against using antipsychotic drugs to prevent severe mental illness', *Journal of Mental Health*, 11: 351–6.

deSwaan, A. (1991) *The Management of Normality*. London: Routledge.

Hiday, V. (1992) 'Coercion in civil commitment: process, preferences and outcome', *International Journal of Law and Psychiatry*, 15: 359–77.

Miller, T.J. and McGlashan, T.H. (2003) 'The risks of not intervening in pre-onset psychotic illness', *Journal of Mental Health*, 12 (4): 345–9.

Rogers, A. (1993) 'Coercion and voluntary admission: an examination of psychiatric patients' views', *Behavioral Sciences and the Law*, 11: 259–67.

Szasz, T.S. (1970) *Ideology and Insanity*. New York: Doubleday.

Szmuckler, G. and Appelbaum, P. (2001) 'Treatment pressures, coercion and compulsion', in G. Thornicroft and G. Szmuckler (eds), *Textbook of Community Psychiatry*. Oxford: Oxford University Press.

The 'Myth of Mental Illness'

***Definition:* The term the 'myth of mental illness' indicates that minds, like economies, can be sick only in a metaphorical sense. People may be frightened, sad, incorrigible or incomprehensible but unless a bodily disease can be proved to underpin these forms of conduct then they are not an indication of mental illness.**

Key points: *• The logic of 'the myth of mental illness' is explained • Critical responses to the notion are outlined.*

The term 'myth of mental illness' was introduced by the American psychiatrist and psychoanalyst Thomas Szasz in the early 1960s. His original paper on the topic in the *American Psychologist* was quickly elaborated as a book with the same title (Szasz, 1961). Szasz has argued that mental illness is a myth because it does not fulfil the criteria, required by scientific medicine, to describe proper illnesses. Originally, he used the terms 'illness' and 'disease' inter-changeably. More recently, in both medicine and medical sociology, the term 'disease' tends to refer to formal professional descriptions of pathology. 'Illness', more typically, refers now to an individual patient's *experience* of being unwell.

Szasz argues that mental illness is a metaphor, rather than a valid description of reality, which is conveniently used by a number of parties. The profession of psychiatry accrues the status of a proper medical specialty by claiming jurisdiction over illness. The State gains from the notion of mental illness because it can delegate lawful powers to medicine for the social control of madness and other forms of social non-conformity (such as personality disorder and drug abuse). Those who do not attract the label of mental illness also gain from the concept because their troublesome fellow citizens can be dealt with by medical paternalism and removed from sight and mind.

Thus Szasz starts with a rather pedantic conceptual point (about the nature of true illnesses) but he quickly moves into a bold form of social and ethical analysis about madness and the role of psychiatry in society, particularly as an agent of social control. He also discusses the history of societal reactions to non-conformity. He concludes that the modern mental patient occupies the same devalued, oppressed and stigmatized role as witches did in the Middle Ages.

Szasz starts with a traditional medical assumption that diseases require that *both* signs and symptoms must be present in an individual to warrant any confident diagnosis. Because psychiatry in its description of functional mental illness *only uses* symptoms (what people say and do) and lacks clear evidence of signs (evidence of bodily abnormality) it is on very weak or even fraudulent grounds as a medical specialty.

The very fact that the medical speciality of psychiatry restricts its own description to mental *illness* (not disease) tends to support Szasz's point that psychiatric diagnosis is based primarily on the patient's experience and conduct.

These four main points summarize what Szasz means, in his argument about the myth of mental illness:

1 He argues that diseases of the brain, which lead to marked changes in thinking and behaviour (for example tertiary syphilis or alcoholic psychosis) are just that – diseases of the brain with psychological consequences. These, he says, should be called proper neurological diseases;
2 By contrast, where a diagnosis starts and finishes *only* with examples of thoughts and action, which others do not understand or do not approve of, then unless a biological cause can be unequivocally demonstrated in the person, then they are not really ill. Hence, to call a person 'mentally ill' is to deploy a metaphor dressed up as a fact. Szasz argues that a mind can only be sick in a metaphorical sense – like an economy or a society;
3 For Szasz, psychiatry's codification of non-conformity as 'mental illness', is thus a logical error. The error then leads to and justifies, for its users and sympathizers, a political scandal and a moral outrage; the coercive control of madness under the guise of medical beneficence and paternalism;
4 By describing mental illness as a 'myth', Szasz does not imply that people are not sad, mad or frightened. His point is that these are ways of being, or 'problems of living', not symptoms of illness. By keeping an open mind about their nature, we may find different ways of

making sense of them. Alternatively, sometimes they may simply remain mysterious. Szasz expresses a preference to interpret 'problems of living' as games or communications, with particular situated meanings for a person in their inter-personal context and life as a whole.

An implication of Szasz's argument is that if a clear set of biological signs of say 'schizophrenia' were ever found, it should then be classified as a true biological disease or illness. Until then, according to Szasz, all functional psychiatric diagnoses, like 'schizophrenia', 'bi-polar disorder', 'depression' and so on should be deemed unscientific and invalid. Psychiatry makes sporadic claims that brain abnormalities can indeed be demonstrated in those with functional diagnoses. However, these claims have been varied, inconsistent and even contradictory. Moreover, cause and effect have never been proven. For example, a detected change in brain biochemistry in a patient could be a *cause* of psychotic symptoms or it could be a *consequence* of stress or the patient's drug treatment.

The provocative position of Szasz has attracted both enthusiastic supporters and indignant critics. Despite being a professor of psychiatry he has repeatedly attacked modern psychiatric theory and practice, and reactions from his colleagues have been varied. From fury or exasperation, many simply ignore him and so cast him beyond the pale. For example, many standard texts in psychiatry significantly omit allusions to his work (e.g. Nicholi, 1999). Silent denial characterizes these texts. Other texts (wrongly) depict the position about the 'myth of mental illness', as being external to the profession, as a form of 'anti-psychiatric' *sociological* attack (e.g. Gelder et al., 2001). This may seek to move the problem of psychiatric knowledge to an envious or hostile enemy without.

Some psychiatrists listen to the attack but still come to the conclusion that the symptom presentation of patients indicates that they are 'obviously mentally ill'. Others argue that while psychiatry may be over-reliant on symptoms, this is also true of physical medicine at times. For example, some conditions like multiple sclerosis are difficult to diagnose. Some diagnoses of reported bodily symptoms have unknown or questionable bodily signs. A reported headache (a symptom) might be a result of muscle tension, a brain tumour or temporary de-hydration. In other words, an over reliance on functional symptoms does not neatly mark off psychiatry from other medical specialties.

Another academic reaction to the work of Szasz has been the argument that *all* illness represent forms of deviance, as it leads to rule breaking or role failure (Sedgwick, 1980). This sociological re-framing of illness as deviance from norms is conceded in Szasz's original article but he still argues that we can come to a stable, democratic and scientific consensus about bodily norms. By contrast, social norms shift over time and place, and policies about their violation are subject to the whims of the powerful in society. As a result, Szasz argues that we would be wise to treat psychiatry and its activity in a different way to the rest of medicine.

His case is supported by the fact that mental illness is treated in a uniquely coercive manner in most modern societies. It is very rare for people with physical illnesses to be controlled coercively by medicine on behalf of State and society. By contrast, it is common for mentally ill patients to have their liberty taken from them without trial and for their bodies to be forcibly interfered with. While detained, patients may also be subject to solitary confinement at the discretion of staff ('seclusion'). These daily realities in mental health services do give substance to Szasz's original concerns about the peculiar character of psychiatric diagnosis and the nature of the treatments the profession typically prescribes.

A final point to note about the gauntlet thrown down by Szasz is that it has probably contributed to more recent demands and criticisms from mental health service users about terminology. The use of 'mental distress', as a preferred alternative to 'mental illness', is an example. Even the more cautious tendency of writers about (rather than within) psychiatry to talk of 'people with a *diagnosis* of mental illness' (rather than 'people *with* mental illness') probably reflects the legacy of Szasz and his claim about the 'myth of mental illness'. It suggests that we can be confident that psychiatric diagnosis regularly occurs but not necessarily that it is legitimate, meaningful or valid.

REFERENCES

Gelder, M., Mayou, R. and Cowen, P. (2001) *Shorter Oxford Textbook of Psychiatry*. Oxford: Oxford University Press.

Nicholi, A.M. (ed.) (1999) *The Harvard Guide to Psychiatry*. Harvard, MA: Belknap.

Sedgwick, P. (1980) *PsychoPolitics*. London: Pluto Press.

Szasz, T.S. (1961) *The Myth of Mental Illness: Foundations of a Theory of Personal Conduct*. New York: Harper & Row.

Eugenics

Definition: Eugenics proposes that human society can be improved by limiting or eliminating the transmission of proved or assumed defective genes.

Key points: • *The history of eugenics is summarized in relation to people with mental health problems* • *Implications for psychiatry and psychology are discussed.*

The profession of psychiatry emerged in the mid-nineteenth century, when the eugenic movement was becoming respectable in both Europe and North America. This was also a time when the founders of differential psychology (the academic basis for testing intelligence and personality in clinical psychology today) began to incorporate eugenic ideas into psychological theories.

In the shadow of the well-documented Nazi genocide is a less well-known policy; the 'mercy killing', by German medical practitioners, of those deemed to constitute 'life devoid of meaning'. The latter term was used to describe patients with any physical or mental incapacity, who were considered to be both a life-long burden on social efficiency and a long-term genetic threat to society. The 'involuntary euthanasia' of psychiatric patients, and other disabled people, was the last point in a collusive relationship between the Nazis and the German Doctors' Association. This started with a shared enthusiasm for the voluntary sterilization of mentally and physically disabled people. This progressed to a policy of involuntary sterilization and culminated in the programme of extermination – enacted not in the Polish death camps but in German hospitals. The policy progression indicated that a eugenic position was common in respectable professional bodies in European society, during the first part of the twentieth century (Meyer, 1988).

The racial focus of political groups like the Nazis was only a variant of the eugenic position. Prior to this right-wing deviation, many left-leaning political theorists advocated eugenic ideas. These focussed on the sexual segregation of groups deemed to be a social problem and on increased birth control to limit the growth of the lowest classes.

A core assumption of eugenics was that human society could be improved by regulating the genetic make up of the population. A corollary of this was that some groups were assumed to be particular threats to this programme of social improvement, especially those deemed to be physically or psychologically imperfect. At the turn of the twentieth century, a common assumption in the educated classes of Europe and North America was that a 'tainted gene pool' existed, which could manifest itself in a range of deviant conduct – madness, epilepsy, idiocy, prostitution, alcoholism and criminality (Forsythe, 1990; Marshall, 1990). Thus, the social problems associated with poverty were not seen as ones of political and economic inequality. Instead, they were viewed as outcomes of degeneracy in those living in destitute conditions.

An indication of the mainstream policy influence of eugenic thinking, continuing well into the twentieth century in Britain, was the report to the government of the Wood Committee. It signalled that the racial focus of Nazism was by no means unique. This official British report talked of the need to prevent the 'racial disaster of mental deficiency'. The latter was considered to be 'the last stage of the inheritance of degeneracy' (HMSO, 1929). Around this time, a whole range of social reform activities in Europe and North America, including the birth control and mental hygiene movements, as well as programmes to sterilize psychiatric patients and those with learning disabilities, reflected eugenic ideas.

With specific regard to development of the mental health professions alongside a cultural norm of racism and eugenics, Fernando (1991) noted the following:

- Psychiatry and psychology incorporated ideas from Darwin, Spencer and Galton. Spencer considered that 'primitive races' had minds like the children of white people. Galton, a founder of eugenics (and the study of individual differences in human psychology), considered that many black people were 'half-witted'. Pearson, a student of Galton and creator of several statistical methods, developed in early academic psychology and still used today, considered that the extermination of 'inferior' races was a logical extension of the evolutionary process. Another example of a eugenic assumption relates to 'Mongolism'. John Langdon Down – hence 'Down's Syndrome' – considered the condition as evidence that idiots were racial 'throwbacks' in the civilized and intellectually superior races;

- These negative assumptions about non-white European stock were also found in prestigious North American psychology texts. For example, Stanley Hall, the founding editor of the *American Journal of Psychology*, considered that the native American 'Indians' or 'Aborigines' were immature and driven by feelings rather than rationality;
- Freud considered that 'primitive' people had less super-ego control (conscience and ideal goals) than white people. Jung was even more elaborate in his theorizing that different racial groups had specific psychological qualities different from one another. His ideas gave comfort to the racist political belief system of the Nazis but the claim that Jung had fascist sympathies remains contentious – see Noll (1997).

A remaining question relates to the current resonance of eugenic ideas within the culture of mental health professionals. The strong biological determinism, which makes a link between madness and the defective genetic make up of patients, still dominates modern psychiatry. This form of determinism was central to the bids for scientific legitimacy by the psychiatric profession in the nineteenth century, and it continued to resonate in the next (Dowbiggin, 1985). There is a traceable link between this dominant current genetic model of madness and eugenically inspired psychiatric research.

The main connection between current psychiatric thought and Nazi eugenics is the work of Eliot Slater (Gottesman and McGuffin, 1996). Slater had worked in Munich since 1934 with the eugenicist psychiatrists Ernst Rudin and Franz Kallman on twin studies started there by Luxemberger (1928). After the war, Rudin was found guilty at the de-Nazification tribunal at Nuremberg. Kallman emigrated to the USA and Slater returned to his native London and propagated the pre-war Munich position about the genetic determination of mental disorders (Slater and Cowie, 1971). Kallman's twin study samples continued to be used as evidence for the genetic determination of schizophrenia in post-war Anglo-American psychiatry, through the work of Slater and his students and collaborators. This research is still cited and endorsed today in psychiatric textbooks.

To conclude, although eugenic ideas may now seem to be outmoded and discredited, they have three forms of recent relevance. First, the current orthodoxy within psychiatry that madness is genetically pre-programmed can be traced, in large part, to eugenicist research during the Nazi period. Second, much of the current personality and intelligence testing in clinical psychology is traceable to a form of late Victorian psychology (the 'psychology of individual differences' or 'differential psychology'), which was promoted by the English eugenicists Francis Galton and Karl Pearson. They started a tradition, at University College London, of psychometric testing to be developed by Spearman, Burt and Eysenck. This tradition informs many of the psychometric tests used today by clinical psychologists (Pilgrim and Treacher, 1992). Third, many of the recent ethical and political debates about euthanasia, genetic counselling, abortion, cloning and in vitro fertilization resonate with those for and against a eugenic position. For example, abortion in the wake of detected foetal abnormality is not only opposed by some religious groups, it also offends many in the disability movement.

See also: *causes and constructs; functional and organic mental illnesses; learning disability.*

REFERENCES

Dowbiggin, I. (1985) 'Degeneration and hereditarianism in French mental medicine 1840–90: psychiatric theory as ideological adaptation', in W.F. Bynum, R. Porter and M. Shepherd (eds), *The Anatomy of Madness (Volume I)*. London: Tavistock.

Fernando, S. (1991) *Mental Health, Race and Culture*. Basingstoke: Macmillan.

Forsythe, B. (1990) 'Mental and social diagnosis and the English Prison Commission 1914–1939', *Social Policy and Administration*, 24 (3): 237–53.

Gottesman, I.I. and McGuffin, P. (1996) 'Eliot Slater and the birth of psychiatric genetics in Great Britain', in H. Freeman and G.E. Berrios (eds), *150 Years of British Psychiatry (Volume II)*. London: Athlone.

HMSO (1929) *Report of the Wood Committee on Mental Deficiency*. London: HMSO.

Luxemberger, H. (1928) 'Vorlaufiger Bericht über psychiatrische Serienuntersuchungen an Zwillingen', *Zieshcrift fur die gesamte Neurologie und Psychiatrie*, 116: 297–326.

Marshall, R. (1990) 'The genetics of schizophrenia', in R.P. Bentall (ed.), *Reconstructing Schizophrenia*. London: Routledge.

Meyer, J.E. (1988) 'The fate of the mentally ill during the Third Reich', *Psychological Medicine*, 18: 575–81.

Noll, R. (1997) *The Aryan Christ: the Secret Life of Carl Gustav Jung*. New York: Random House.

Pilgrim, D. and Treacher, A. (1992) *Clinical Psychology Observed*. London: Routledge.

Slater, E. and Cowie, V. (1971) *The Genetics of Mental Disorders*. London: Oxford University Press.

Corruption of Care

***Definition:* 'By this is meant the fact that primary aims of care – the cure or alleviation of suffering – have become subordinate to what are essentially secondary aims, such as the creation and preservation of order, quiet and cleanliness . . .' (Martin, 1984).**

Key points: • *The main features of 'scandal hospitals' are described* • *The potential role of corruption of care in prompting hospital run down is discussed.*

The entry on malpractice discusses this phenomenon at the level of the individual practitioner. In this entry, a higher level description is given about the ways that care *systems* can fail. The term 'corruption of care' was coined by John Martin (1984) in his book *Hospital in Trouble*. Martin was interested in reviewing the conclusions of reports on recurrent neglect and abuse in mental illness and mental handicap hospitals (the terminology of the time). He looked at a period between 1965 and 1980 and drew out some overall conclusions or lessons:

- *Chronicity of client group* A characteristic of these hospitals was that they dealt with long-term patient populations. The chronicity of the groups of people with learning disabilities or with a range of long-term mental health problems meant that they were socially devalued and voiceless. It also meant that they were unrewarding to the staff responsible for them. The fact that the patient groups were diverse (in terms of diagnosis) suggests that problems of neglect and abuse could be largely accounted for by the failure of policy makers, managers and practitioners to respond efficiently and humanely to chronic deviance;
- *Geographical isolation* The policy in the Victorian period was to build large institutions in rural places or on the outskirts of urban areas. These places were typically marked off by perimeter walls. Their distance from others in society meant that lay visiting was infrequent

and in controlled periods. Ordinary external scrutiny was therefore limited. Another aspect of geographical isolation was that it was common for staff to be drawn from a relatively closed local population. Staff could work all of their lives in one place and their children could repeat this process;

- *Ward isolation* The hospitals were so large that they were divided into many separate units or wards. A feature of 'scandal hospitals' was that they manifested a 'fiefdom mentality'. That is, those running the individual wards enjoyed a sense of separateness and autonomy, with senior staff having the discretion to use their personal power as they wished. A neglectful norm could then readily develop. Staff could ignore patients and their needs and relate predominantly to one another instead. They could ensure that daily ward routines were attended to without reference to the needs of patients;
- *Personal staff isolation* An extension of ward isolation was that the wards had long periods with low staffing levels. A few staff members might be left alone to look after large numbers of difficult to manage or unrewarding patients for long periods of time;
- *Medical isolation* A feature of hospitals with problems was that medical staff would be distant from ward activity. Consultants would visit wards infrequently. The more unrewarding and chronic the group, the more this tendency occurred. As with infrequent lay scrutiny from visitors, this meant that the beginnings of bad practice were not spotted by outsiders to the daily ward environment;
- *Intellectual isolation* Because staff might work on wards for many years on end with little or no updated training, they had a tendency to become isolated from professional knowledge. This meant that they lost touch with changes in both technical knowledge and professional ethics;
- *Privacy* While neglect was typically an insidious process, whereby standards of care might deteriorate over time, quite openly, within a ward fiefdom, abuse was a different matter. The latter (which was typically about physical mistreatment) required conditions of privacy, where one or two staff members were alone with a victim or victims. Ward and personal isolation, noted above, created the conditions for this possibility of privacy.

Martin's account of organizational failure can itself be placed in a political and historical context. The history of the Victorian hospitals involved mental health nurses coming from a legacy of manhandling. That is, the psychiatric branch of nursing, which became professionalized in the twentieth century, was not connected to the medical or physical branch of the profession. The latter, championed by Florence Nightingale, was middle class, genteel and female. By contrast, the asylum attendants of the nineteenth century were male and working class, with many of them moving in and out of other forms of unskilled manual work (Carpenter, 1980). Nightingale and her successors actively resisted this group entering the profession of nursing for many years. Thus, the roots of hospital-based mental health nursing were characterized by a norm of physical (and of necessity) rough handling.

Another contributory feature of the historical context was the use of physical restraint and treatment. This is a medical not a nursing feature. Alienists, mad-doctors and the early psychiatrists established a norm of bodily interference. Mechanical restraints, such as straightjackets, were common in the asylum system. Cold compresses and dunking in cold baths were often medically prescribed in response to agitated or disruptive patient behaviour well into the twentieth century.

The bio-medical preference for medicinal responses meant that it became common for patients to be restrained and forcibly injected with tranquillizers. This increasing practice, during the late twentieth century, at times led to the death of patients. These professional norms about physical interference were only a short distance away from physical abuse, with 'use' and 'abuse' being difficult to distinguish. Once physical interference became a norm, then treatment, the pragmatic management of disruption or threat and punishment were easily jumbled in the minds and actions of staff.

By and large, these scandals appear to be a thing of the past (at least in those countries with a programme of large hospital closure). However, many of the features of systemic isolation still apply in two senses. First, with re-institutionalization (the tendency for chronic cases now to reside in long-term small nursing homes or private hospitals) the corruption of care remains possible. Second, in Britain and other countries, which closed most of their large mental hospitals, forensic facilities are retained. For example, in Britain we still have four large high-security hospitals (Ashworth, Broadmoor, Carstairs and Rampton). The final report discussed by Martin was about abuse at Rampton Hospital. During the 1980s and 1990s further official inquiries into neglect and abuse emerged in the high-security hospitals (previously called the Special Hospital system) (Kaye and Franey, 1998). Some of these were prompted by the death in seclusion of patients, who had been manhandled and forcibly tranquillized. Black patients were disproportionately represented in these deaths.

Given the public shock and professional shame created by scandals, involving the neglect or abuse of psychiatric patients, it is tempting to ascribe particular causal powers to the inquiries summarized by Martin. They could be seen as an important political determinant of hospital closure policy ('desegregation'). However, this would be misleading for three reasons.

First, competing accounts of desegregation do not place a large emphasis on official inquiries into maltreatment but suggest other factors, such as technical changes in care and cost (Busfield, 1986; Rogers and Pilgrim, 2005).

Second, some of the recent inquiry reports explicitly recommended hospital closure but no action then ensued. This was the case, not once but twice, during the 1990s, in relation to Ashworth Hospital, which remains open (though its patient numbers have been reduced).

Third, the wider critique of institutional psychiatry (hospital-based, dehumanizing and bio-medically orientated), known as 'anti-psychiatry', acquired little governmental credibility in most Western countries (except Italy). As a consequence, it had little influence on mainstream governmental decision making about mental health policy. Basically, States abandoned large hospitals only when they were politically and economically ready to do so, not because conditions in them were scandalous. After all, they had been highly oppressive places for over a hundred years. With good cause they were feared by those on the outside and certainly suffered by those on the inside – hence the concept of being a 'psychiatric survivor'. Although injected tranquillization created a new source of patient death in the last quarter of the twentieth century (Kellam, 1987), from the outset the asylums were a threat to life. In the mid-nineteenth century, when the asylum system was burgeoning, around 40% of admissions to hospital were soon dead (Russell, 1985).

Together these three points reinforce a fundamental and persistent aspect of mental health policy: it has been driven, by and large, by the need for social order. This means that the social control of deviance, if necessary with the use of staff force and without care for the human rights of patients, has been central to government concerns. This conclusion suggests that inquiries investigating *organizational failures* might also be recording the dark side of a *political success* in controlling incorrigible deviance. If this conclusion is correct, then it is unlikely that the 'corruption of care' will disappear in the foreseeable future.

See also: *segregation; 'anti-psychiatry'; malpractice; forensic mental health services.*

REFERENCES

Busfield, J. (1986) *Managing Madness*. London: Hutchinson.

Carpenter, M. (1980) 'Asylum nursing before 1914: a chapter in the history of nursing', in C. Davies (ed.), *Re-writing Nursing History*. London: Croom Helm.

Kaye, C. and Franey, A. (eds) (1998) *Managing High Security Psychiatric Care*. London: Jessica Kingsley.

Kellam, A.M.P. (1987) 'The neuroleptic syndrome, so called: a survey of the world literature', *British Journal of Psychiatry*, 150: 752–9.

Martin, J.P. (1984) *Hospitals in Trouble*. Oxford: Blackwell.

Rogers, A. and Pilgrim, D. (2005) *A Sociology of Mental Health and Illness (Third Edition)*. Maidenhead: Open University Press.

Russell, R. (1985) 'The lunacy profession and its staff in the second half of the nineteenth century, with special reference to the West Riding Lunatic Asylum', in W.F. Byum, R. Porter and M. Shepherd (eds), *The Anatomy of Madness (Volume III)*. London: Tavistock.

Malpractice

***Definition:* Malpractice refers to improper professional behaviour. It includes wilful neglect and any form of exploitation of the client to gratify the practitioner.**

Key points: *• Malpractice in health care is discussed • The particular significance of malpractice for people with mental health problems is highlighted • Responses to the phenomenon of malpractice from different interest groups are summarized.*

Malpractice is one part of a series of ways in which mental health professionals might fail their clients. Both physical and psychological mental health interventions are researched under ideal conditions of randomized controlled trials in which optimal practice is being observed. In routine service provision or in private practice the chances of sub-optimal professional practice are multiple.

First, practitioners may make mistakes. Errors of judgement and memory are ordinary human failings and so all health and social care professionals are thus susceptible, some of the time to this risk.

Second, practitioners may be careless and demonstrate poor practice. For example, they may keep poor records or they may be lax in breaking the rule of strict confidentiality. As with errors, carelessness may be unintentional but sometimes this is not the case. Also, carelessness may be a product of organizational failures not just individual shortcomings (or the latter may flow from the former). For example, practitioners may be poorly trained or their employers may not provide the time and resources for them to keep their practice up to date and well supervised. Thus when negligence does occur, there may be uncertainty about whether it is a moral or organizational failure (or both).

Third, the practitioner may deliberately exploit clients. In formal terms, this third area is definitely about malpractice but its ethical and legal status is not neatly separable from wilful negligence.

In mental health services errors and poor practice are dealt with mainly by a process of audit. That is 'critical incidents' or 'near misses' are routinely logged and discussed by service managers and corrective action considered and at times implemented. For example, error rates in the administration of drugs by nurses can be monitored and new safeguards introduced. Mistakes, carelessness and poor practice are mainly dealt with as organizational failures, although occasionally they may lead to disciplinary action against individual practitioners.

The shift from a framework, which mainly emphasizes *organizational determinism*, to one which places *moral culpability* centre stage is important. A problem about the whole area of bad practice is that lay people and professionals do not always agree about the balance to be struck between these two. This has led to the anomalous position of health care organizations emphasizing the need for a 'no blame' culture, while at the same time using internal and external disciplinary mechanisms to make poor practitioners individually accountable for their actions. (This contradiction reflects a deeper ambivalence in modern society about determinism and human agency. The common uncertainty about how to understand and respond to professional neglect and abuse is symptomatic of this wider ambivalence.)

The peculiar ways in which people with mental health problems are open to abuse are discussed in the section on the 'Corruption of Care' but here it should be noted that they are particularly vulnerable to exploitation for a number of reasons:

- Some people with mental health problems may lack the capacity to appreciate that they are being exploited;
- Their primary mental health problems may lead to a highly dependent stance in relation to professionals. For example, patients who are highly anxious may become childlike in their dependency on fellow adults, including mental health professionals. In another example, some patients are highly suggestible. Histrionic patients are particularly vulnerable in this regard;
- Even if a person with a mental health problem properly reflects on abusive professional action and proceeds to complain legitimately, their mental state may undermine their credibility in the eyes of third party adjudicators. A variant of this is that even if the latter are credulous about a patient's account, the patient may lack the confidence that they will be believed;
- The tradition of individual casework, in counselling and psychotherapy, sets up the physical conditions in which abuse may be more likely. This has resonances with other health care scenarios, where unchaperoned intimate meetings occur. For example, most publicized cases of sexual malpractice involve GPs, psychological therapists or gyneacologists. This is not to say that privacy causes exploitation – it is a necessary but not a sufficient condition. Most health care workers do not use this condition of privacy to exploit their clients, but the exploitative minority is not insignificant. Estimates of psychological therapists who admit, in anonymous surveys, to sexual relationships with one or more clients varies from 4–8%. This may be an underestimate, as even in anonymous surveys professionals are likely to under-report malpractice. In the USA over half of the malpractice actions against mental health workers are about sexual contact with clients.

Ideas about correcting or minimizing malpractice vary. Some argue for example that psychotherapy has such a poor track record in relation to financial, emotional, physical and sexual abuse that it should be avoided at all costs. The argument for this radical suggestion is developed in *Against Therapy* by Jeffrey Masson (1992). Users who have survived malpractice argue for more stringent and quicker judgements about exploitative professionals, once a complaint is lodged. The professional response has tended to emphasize more effective supervision and training (continued professional development). Governmental responses have focused more on legal regulation. There are international differences in the latter regard. For example, in many states in the USA sexual malpractice is criminalized but in the UK it is not dealt with under criminal law but only as a professional disciplinary matter.

A major challenge faced by mental health professional bodies is that an emphasis on extensive training, supervision and legal registration (the traditional web of safeguards offered to the public) has not always been persuasive to disaffected service users. Abusive therapists who are exposed are often found to be well-qualified and appropriately registered to practice. Moreover, the disciplinary proceedings used when complaints are used are often protracted and distressing. Even when a practitioner is expelled for malpractice ('struck off'), this is rarely a lifelong ban. These processes can give the impression that professional interests, rightly or wrongly, are privileged when legitimate complaints are made by abused clients.

The question of physical abuse is complicated. For example, mental health workers are lawfully permitted to impose physical treatments on dissenting bodies. In any other circumstance, this would be common assault. By contrast, physical contact is considered to be unethical in codes of practice governing psychological therapies. (Even here there are exceptions, as in the case of 'body therapies'.)

Emotional abuse too is not always easy to define and demonstrate in the quasi-judicial setting of disciplinary proceedings triggered by client complaints. In a very broad sense, any psychological therapist must be gaining some emotional gratification in their work. They listen privately to one after another problematic personal account of others, week in week out for years on end. This unusual professional lifestyle must be sustained by some personal gain for the therapist begging a question: at what point is a therapist's emotional needs being privileged over their client's?

The notion of financial exploitation is even more open to interpretation because of the norms of private practice in mental health work. Some forms of psychotherapy are long-term and so cumulatively take large quantities of money from paying clients. Also, value for money is a consumer judgement. But the latter in some forms of psychotherapy is simply seen as one of many symbolic communications to discuss in the therapy. The client who pays late or complains about paying is not simply seen as a rational customer with consumer rights. Instead, these communications about the fee are simply material to interpret, along with others about the person and their life. In this context, financial exploitation is difficult to define in clear terms. Given these complexities in relation to the physical, emotional and financial norms of therapist action, it is not surprising that sexual malpractice tends to be investigated more (both in disciplinary proceedings and in research).

See also: *risks to and from people with mental health problems; psychological interventions; biological interventions; coercion; corruption of care; capacity and culpability.*

FURTHER READING

Bersoff, D.N. (1995) *Ethical Conflicts in Psychology*. Washington, DC: American Psychological Association.

Lifson, L.E. and Simon, R.I. (eds) (1998) *The Mental Health Practitioner and the Law*. London: Harvard University Press.

Masson, J. (1992) *Against Therapy*. London: Fontana.

Palmer Barnes, F. (1998) *Complaints and Grievances in Psychotherapy*. London: Routledge.

Pilgrim, D. and Guinan, P. (1999) 'From mitigation to culpability: rethinking the evidence about therapist sexual abuse', *European Journal of Counselling, Psychotherapy and Health*, 2 (2): 153–68.

Capacity and Culpability

***Definition:* 'Capacity' is a legal term referring to the ability of a person to make sound rational judgements. A closely related notion is that of culpability – the extent to which a wrong doer is deemed to be responsible for their actions. Both involve notions of personal awareness and personal responsibility. They imply autonomous human action.**

Key points: *• Considerations about mental disorder and personal capacity are discussed • Legal considerations about the culpability of mentally disordered offenders are outlined.*

A vexed question for all concerned in mental health policy and practice relates to human agency – the quality most of us have, as we mature, to reflect on our actions and anticipate in advance their consequences. As the above definition indicates, it is common for judgements to be made by third parties that some patients are incapable of understanding the nature and consequences of their own actions, or the impact of actions of others on them. Also, personal agency may be queried when wrong doing occurs at the hands of people who are deemed to be mentally abnormal. This complexity will be discussed now under a number of points.

- *Capacity as a relative concept* Generally, capacity is attributed to adults but not to children. However, the attribution of personal capacity to a 13-year-old is greater than to a 3-year-old, even though legally both are children. Similarly, a person in the early stages of dementia will be deemed to have more capacity than another in its later stages;
- *Neurological and psychiatric cases* The example of dementia points up a common reason for a person being deemed to lack capacity. Some of the dispute around mental disorder and capacity hinges on the legitimacy of medical diagnoses. In the case of organic mental illnesses – which are true neurological diseases – arguments against paternalism are less strong and less common. Disputes tend to arise in relation to functional psychiatric diagnoses, including personality disorder. Moreover, whether a condition is judged to be organic or functional, then a medical judgement still has to be made about the *extent* to which a person's disorder might impair their capacity;
- *Judgements about incapacity have consequences* Once the judgement is made about lack of capacity then consequences flow. For example, if a person is deemed to lack capacity then third parties are expected to make decisions on their behalf. An example here might be of a parent deciding that a young adult with learning disabilities, who is sexually active, should be sterilized. The operation then proceeds with the parents' consent. Less dramatic examples are of third parties receiving pension payments on behalf of a dementing patient. In the case of patients with functional diagnoses, such as schizophrenia, third parties (relatives, social workers and psychiatrists) may frequently negotiate desirable outcomes on their behalf. In all of these cases, medical ethicists tend to use the notion of 'impaired autonomy', rather than the legal notion of 'capacity'. This takes us to the next point;
- *Impaired autonomy is a social judgement* Medical ethics relies for its guidance on principles developed by the philosopher J.S. Mill. He argued that in a civilized society the autonomy of law-abiding citizens should be respected and protected at all times *except* in the cases of

children, the insane and idiots – 'those who are still in a state to require being taken care of by others must be protected against their own actions, as well as against external injury'. This gives the green light for mental health professionals to act in a warranted paternalistic way towards their patients. Indeed, according to Mill, they are *obliged* to act in that way.

Problems arise, though, when disputes are introduced about the *extent* to which a person is deemed to lack capacity and about the *consequences* of restraint. In the first case, anti-paternalists argue that mentally disordered people can and should make judgements on their own behalf. Paternalists argue that they cannot and that doctors are obliged to intervene, as a duty of care. In the second case (about restraint) there is a different dispute. Paternalists argue that a failure to restrain in order to treat, risks a deterioration of the mental disorder. Anti-paternalists argue that (metaphorically) the cure may be worse than the disease. An example here would be of a deluded patient who is coping on their own but, by the agreement of all, is mad or 'suffering from a severe mental illness'. They are detained in hospital involuntarily under the Mental Health Act and forcibly medicated. They lose their accommodation. They lose their liberty. They are put at risk of the adverse effects of anti-psychotic medication. Which is ethically preferable, intervening or letting them be?

Another example is the problem in making decisions about the anorexic patient whose body weight drops to a life threatening level. These patients are not typically psychotic. In all normal respects they are sane and can reason logically. The risk to the self is very high though; should medical intervention be imposed? If so, should it be limited to life-saving nutritional first aid or should it extend to a longer compulsory period of psychiatric detention? If it is the latter for how long?;

- *Inconsistency in decision making about culpability* When it comes to dangerousness to others, rather than to the self, there are examples of inconsistency. For example, some sex offenders are sent to prison. Others are sent to a secure hospital. Inside mental health facilities, psychotic patients who act in an anti-social way are tolerated by staff but those with a diagnosis of personality disorder acting in a similar fashion are not. Both are being treated within a paternalistic medical regime but one group is still deemed to be responsible for their actions and so are treated moralistically and critically, whereas the other is not;

- *Variants of impaired legal culpability* While arguments about capacity are often about the risk of impaired judgement jeopardizing the health or even life of the patient, those about culpability refer to criminal acts against others. In criminal law, for a person to be judged guilty, the court must be satisfied that there was malicious intent on the part of the perpetrator. In the case of the accused not being mentally disordered then an act may be judged to be unintentional or accidental. This may lead to the perpetrator not being tried or being acquitted. Unintended but reckless or negligent acts (such as manslaughter) are lesser crimes than those where 'malice aforethought', 'intention' or '*mens rea*' is evident. For this reason, they tend to lead to less severe sentencing. In the case of British mentally disordered offenders, these decision-making processes may be overridden in a variety of ways.

  First, the perpetrator may not be deemed fit to stand trial – they lack a 'fitness to plead'. In these circumstances, they may be sent to a secure hospital without trial, provided that their role in the offence is clear to the court. If their mental disorder is treatable or recovery emerges naturally with time, then they may be recalled at a later date to face trial.

  Second, whether or not the patient is deemed fit to plead, they may be judged to be 'not guilty by reason of insanity'. When this is the case, then the court, having taken psychiatric advice, decides that the person was sufficiently mentally disordered *at the time of the offence* that they were unaware that their actions were wrong. The insanity defence is more common in some countries than others. It is rare in Britain, where the third contingency is more likely to operate, when a case of homicide is being considered by the court.

  Third, the defence of 'diminished responsibility' can be invoked, when mentally disordered offenders commit murder, but not in the case of other crimes in current English law. The legal term used in this context is suffering from 'abnormality of mind', which does not map neatly on to diagnostic categories preferred by psychiatrists.

  Fourth, the most contentious decision is in relation to temporary loss of reason and intention. This might apply to automatism (crimes committed while sleepwalking) and more commonly but also, more controversially, crimes committed while under the influence of drugs or alcohol. Substance abuse is particularly contentious. On the one hand it is deemed to be a mental disorder. On the other hand in some crimes, such as dangerous driving, the intoxicated driver is typically treated much more harshly, by the courts, than the sober one. When this happens, the presence of a mental disorder, where the offender can demonstrate their long-term substance dependence, does not mitigate the action but the reverse occurs. This is against the trend of general decision making in relation to mentally disordered offenders. However, this does not imply that a hospital 'disposal' by the courts necessarily leads to a lesser period of detention than imprisonment for the perpetrator, merely that the conditions of detention are likely to be more humane.

See also: *substance misuse; learning disability; forensic mental health services.*

FURTHER READING

Dunn, C. (1998) *Ethical Issues in Mental Illness*. London: Ashgate.
Gillon, R. (1997) *Philosophical Medical Ethics*. London: Wiley.
Gunn, J. and Taylor, P. (eds) (1993) *Forensic Psychiatry: Clinical, Legal and Ethical Issues*. London: Butterworth/Heinemann.
Markham, D. (2003) 'Attitudes towards patients with a diagnosis of "borderline personality disorder": social rejection and dangerousness', *Journal of Mental Health*, 12 (6): 595–612.

'Anti-psychiatry'

***Definition:* 'Anti-psychiatry' describes the work of a range of professional critics of orthodox psychiatric theory and practice.**

Key points: *• The character of anti-psychiatry is described • The main themes which connect anti-psychiatry with more recent views from post-psychiatry and the mental health service users' movement are described.*

'Anti-psychiatry' can be heard as a term of hostile contempt from some who defend traditional theory and practice in psychiatry. It may be used resentfully or dismissively about, or against, any idea or person critical of the profession and its norms. Less emotively, it is also used to describe the output of a range of thinkers from a variety of countries in the 1960s, who offered a set of critiques about psychiatry. These included the published work of the psychiatrists Thomas Szasz (USA), Franco Basaglia (Italy), David Cooper (England), Ronald Laing (Scotland), Frantz Fanon (Algeria) and Jacques Lacan (France). Also, some North American sociologists, particularly those promoting labelling theory, contributed to this constellation of ideas, such as Erving Goffman and Thomas Scheff. The work of the French philosopher Michel Foucault also added to the mix, although some of his later ideas fitted less readily. Most of these thinkers are now dead but their criticisms remain influential.

With the exception of David Cooper, none of these luminaries embraced the label of 'anti-psychiatry'. Thomas Szasz actively rejected the term. To him it implied being opposed to *everything* that psychiatry does and so it is logically absurd. As most of those associated with the intellectual leadership of 'anti-psychiatry' were *psychiatrists*, Szasz had a point. By and large though, the label was *about* the critics rather than from them. Despite this ambivalence from the critical group, the label stuck to it – an irony given that the hazards of labelling were central to its critique. The notion of a 'constellation of ideas' is used here neutrally because when the term 'anti-psychiatry' was used by defenders of the profession, there was more than a strong hint of an organized global attack.

In support of this conspiracy theory, it is true that contributors came from all over the world and they often referenced and supported one another's work. However, this trend was inconsistent and the political ideology of the group was mixed. It included liberals like Goffman, Marxists like Cooper, left-leaning humanists like Laing and strident anti-communists like Szasz. Indeed, the latter can be considered a right-wing libertarian because of his consistent hostility to the role of the State, as an enemy of individual freedom and his support for the free market. By contrast, Foucault was a left-wing libertarian and some of his work was out of sync with the strong humanist current in many of the other thinkers. The evidence of attack from different parts of the world probably says more about the vulnerability of psychiatric theory and practice than the conspiratorial motives of its critics. Psychiatry was and remains an easy target of criticism and so its practitioners are understandably wary and weary of being attacked.

The anti-establishment and libertarian culture of the 1960s was also reflected in the fiction of the period, which included themes resonant with the 'anti-psychiatric' position. Examples included Hannah Green's *I Never Promised You a Rose Garden*, Doris Lessing's *Golden Notebooks* and Ken Kesey's *One Flew Over the Cuckoo's Nest.* The latter, starring Jack Nicholson, became an international box-office success at the cinema.

The 'anti-psychiatric' clinicians in diverse ways promoted a radicalized version of psychoanalysis (Lacan, Szasz and Laing were psychoanalysts). Marxist and Weberian social science (Marcuse and Goffman respectively) were influential. Also, the influences of existentialism (Sartre) and phenomenology (Merleu-Ponty) were evident. Laing's work also drew upon Eastern ways, especially Buddhism. By the 1970s, a range of feminist writers began to address 'anti-psychiatric' themes, particularly critiques of the modern family (for example, Kate Millet and Shulamith Firestone), as well as exploring the confluence of psychoanalysis and feminism (for example, Juliet Mitchell).

The summary above does not imply that the 1960s was the first period when psychiatry's knowledge base and role in society had attracted criticism. 'Anti-psychiatry' came in the immediate wake of the publication in 1958 of Barbara Wootton's influential book *Social Science and Social Pathology*. This attacked value judgements masquerading as science in diagnosis and the interfering role of psychiatric professionals. Also, there had been a long tradition, since the early 1920s, of critical theory derived from the work of the Frankfurt School – a range of writers discussing the implications of the confluence of Marxian and Freudian thinking.

There is evidence of the continuing influence of 'anti-psychiatry'. Many disaffected users, who during the 1970s and 1980s began to organize themselves into a new social movement to oppose orthodox psychiatric theory and practice, drew heavily upon 'anti-psychiatric' work. Also, a new generation of 'critical psychiatrists' emerged during the 1990s, which now focuses on very similar concerns to its predecessors. Sometimes this intellectual position, which has been mainly influenced by the work of Michel Foucault and other founders of post-modern social science, is now called 'post-psychiatry'.

Here are a series of critical concerns that connect 'anti-psychiatry', the mental health service users' movement and 'post-psychiatry':

- *The meaning of madness* While the traditional medical view of madness is that it is an illness, probably resulting from a genetically programmed deterioration of the brain, critics query this or offer alternative views. For example, Laing and Cooper were keen to explore the ways in which unintelligible conduct might make sense within a person's social situation (particularly in the family). Similarly, critical service users more recently have organized Hearing Voices groups. These do not pre-judge the meaning of auditory hallucinations, as the pathological by-product of a schizophrenic illness. Instead, people are helped to examine the role of the voices in their particular biographical context. This is a central theme of 'anti-psychiatry'; the shift from patients as examples of an assumed general pathology (say 'schizophrenia') to people with problems requiring individualized forms of understanding;

- *The problem of coercion* Critics of psychiatry have criticized its coercive role. Coercion is rarely used to enforce medical treatment. By contrast, psychiatry uses coercion on a daily basis. Because coercive powers are delegated lawfully to psychiatry, the profession accepts its legitimacy and is often unreflective about its implications. More than that, it takes medical paternalism to its furthest point by emphasizing the doctor's right to treat rather than the patient's right to liberty;
- *The problem of stigmatization* Critics of psychiatry complain that it makes an active contribution to the stigmatization of psychological difference by the use of devaluing diagnoses, such as 'schizophrenia';
- *The problem of social exclusion* A consequence of coercive removal from society and stigmatizing diagnoses is that psychiatric patients have their citizenship undermined. This focus has been less evident since the run down of the old asylum system but newer services are criticized for their bio-medical character and their lack of concern for the advocacy of social inclusion for patients;
- *The psychiatric preoccupation with physical treatments* A final theme in the views of critics is the unimaginative over-use of drug treatments and electro-convulsive therapy (ECT) by psychiatry. The lesser common psychosurgery is a particular focus of opposition but ECT also comes in for recurrent criticism. Campaigns can still be found to outlaw both ECT and psychosurgery. Alternatives suggested by critics range from non-intervention to various forms of psychotherapy.

These themes remain live in current debates about mental health services and the professional priorities of those who work in them. They are also still evident in the demands made for service improvements by local user groups.

See also: *the 'myth of mental illness'; coercion; biological interventions; stigma; mental health service quality.*

FURTHER READING

Basaglia, F. (1968) *L'instituzione negata*. Milan: Einaudi. (For an English summary of his ideas see his chapter in Ingleby, D. (ed.) (1980) *Critical Psychiatry: the Politics of Mental Health*. Harmondsworth: Penguin.)

Clare, A. (1976) *Psychiatry in Dissent*. London: Tavistock.

Cooper, D. (1968) *Psychiatry and Anti-psychiatry*. London: Tavistock.

Fanon, F. (1963) *The Wretched of the Earth*. London: Granada.

Firestone, S. (1970) *The Dialectic of Sex: The Case for Feminist Revolution*. New York: Morrow.

Foucault, M. (1967) *Madness and Civilization*. London: Tavistock.

Goffman, E. (1961) *Asylums*. Harmondsworth: Penguin.

Green, H. (1964) *I Never Promised You a Rose Garden*. New York: Holt.

Kesey, K. (1962) *One Flew Over the Cuckoo's Nest*. New York: Viking.

Kotowitz, Z. (1997) *R.D. Laing and the Paths of Anti-psychiatry*. London: Routledge.

Laing, R.D. (1967) *The Politics of Experience and the Bird of Paradise*. Harmondsworth: Penguin.

Lessing, D. (1962) *The Golden Notebook*. New York: Simon and Schuster.

Millet, K. (1970) *Sexual Politics*. New York: Doubleday.

Mitchell, J. (1971) *Women's Estate*. New York: Pantheon.

Roth, M. (1973) 'Psychiatry and its critics', *British Journal of Psychiatry*, 122: 174–6.

Scheff, T. (1966) *Being Mentally Ill: a Sociological Theory*. New York: Aldine.

Sedgwick, P. (1980) *PsychoPolitics*. London: Pluto Press.

Szasz, T.S. (1971) *The Manufacture of Madness*. London: Routledge.

Wing, J. (1978) *Reasoning About Madness*. Oxford: Oxford University Press.

Wootton, B. (1958) *Social Science and Social Pathology*. London: Routledge and Kegan Paul.

Labelling Theory

***Definition:* Labelling theory is a sociological approach to the study of deviance, which emphasizes the ways in which rule breaking and role failure are maintained by the reactions of others. For this reason, labelling theory is also known as 'societal reaction theory'.**

Key points: *• The strengths and weaknesses of labelling theory are described • The more recent development of 'modified labelling theory' is outlined.*

Labelling theory developed from one wing of the Chicago School of Sociology, 'symbolic interactionism', which understands society by studying the ways in which humans exchange meanings in their interactions. Within this general approach, labelling theory focuses on the reaction of others to deviance. It accepts that the origin of *primary deviance* (say, being mentally disordered) may include a variety of biological, psychological and social causes. The focus though for labelling theorists is mainly on the maintenance and amplification of *secondary deviance*. The reactions of others shape the latter. Others may ignore or focus on deviant conduct, depending on a range of social contingencies.

Yarrow et al. (1955) found that the wives of men eventually labelled as schizophrenic ignored and rationalized symptoms for varying periods of time before seeking help. Rosenhan (1973) showed that 'pseudo-patients' were admitted to psychiatric facilities for simply reporting hearing the words 'empty', 'hollow' and 'thud'. In all other respects, they behaved rationally. The psychiatric staff recorded all of their behaviour, as if it was indicative of mental illness.

In these studies, there was confusion about the significant labellers. For Scheff (1966) it was psychiatrists. For Goffman (1961) it was the family, psychiatrists and staff in the mental hospital. However, there was an agreement that labelling irrevocably alters the person's identity and social status. Once a person is seen to have lost their reason, then their credibility is permanently undermined (Garfinkel, 1956). Their old identity is cast off and a new one takes its place (a 'status degradation ceremony'). Part of such a process then leads to the labelled person internalizing the new identity ascribed to them. This is then maintained by self-labelling and the expectations of others.

After the 1960s labelling theory fell out of favour because of a number of criticisms:

- Gove (1975) argued that it understates the underlying power of the causes of primary deviance. Moreover, Gove claimed that labelling has the positive consequence of giving patients access to help to reduce their deviance;
- If lay people play such an important role in deviance amplification then we would expect everyday stereotypes of mental illness to match psychiatric diagnoses. However, Jones and Cochrane (1981) found that stereotypes conform very poorly to what psychiatrists diagnose in their work. The typical stereotype of a wild deranged patient is wholly inaccurate. The most common diagnosis of 'depression' tends not to be mentioned in lay stereotypes of mental illness. Also Rosenhan's

pseudo-patients did not go on to actually take on the role of psychiatric patients after their discharge from hospital;

- Labelling theory does not really provide us with a clear picture of what the salient contingencies are that make the difference between deviance being ignored or being ascribed.

On this last point, some circumstances do seem to predict the ascription of mental illness. Women are more likely to be labelled than men in lay networks. Also, the greater the personal gap between labellers and the potentially labelled (in relation to race, culture, gender and class), the greater the chances of mental illness being ascribed and the more negative the label (Horwitz, 1982).

Despite the demise in popularity of labelling theory in the 1970s, more recent favourable appraisals have emphasized the substantial evidence for labelling theory, albeit in a modified form. Link and Phelan (1999) have drawn attention to a number of studies, which clearly demonstrate the negative effects of labelling:

- Some studies indicate that disvalued social statuses, such as prostitution, epilepsy, alcoholism, and drug abuse form a hierarchy of stigma, with mental illness being near to the bottom (e.g. Skinner et al., 1995);
- Some experimental studies also show that knowledge of a person's psychiatric history predicts social rejection and that these tendencies start in childhood (e.g. Harris et al., 1990);
- Surveys of the general public show that fear of violence and the need to keep a social distance diminish with increasing contact with people with a psychiatric diagnosis (Alexander and Link, 2003);
- Some studies, even at the time that labelling theory was losing its popularity demonstrated that a psychiatric history reduced a person's access to housing and employment (e.g. Farina and Felner, 1973).

These types of finding have led to 'modified labelling theory'. Link and Phelan (1999) confirmed two main findings in a series of studies. First, provided that best practice is offered in mental health services, people with mental health problems can derive positive benefits (supporting Gove's claim about the positive opportunity created by labelling). Second, whether or not specialist mental health services have positive or negative effects (a function of their range of quality) independent effects of stigma and social rejection persist in the community.

The theory Link and colleagues have developed to account for this second finding, relates not to direct prejudicial action by others (the 'classical' position of labelling theory) but by a shared cultural expectation. The latter entails mental illness leading to suspicion, loss of credibility and social rejection. All parties, including and *especially* the person who *develops* a mental health problem, share this assumption from childhood. Consequently, the patient enters, or considers entering, interactions with others with this shared negative assumption. Non-patients also expect patients to be expecting social distance. This shared view then leads to both parties lacking confidence in their interaction, creating a self-fulfilling prophecy. The patient keeps their distance and the non-patient expects and lets this occur. Subsequently, this creates social disability and isolation in the patient.

Modified labelling theory is also supported by the work of Thoits (1985), who noted that classical labelling theory was preoccupied with involuntary relationships, whereas most consultations for mental health problems occur voluntarily, mainly in primary care services. Thoits demonstrates how we learn from a young age to self monitor emotional deviance.

For example, we begin to learn when it is appropriate to be happy, sad or fearful. Consequently, we also can identify in ourselves when our emotional conduct might be considered inappropriate by others. Thoits describes this as a shared awareness of the compliance with, or transgression of, 'feeling rules'. For example, the phobic patient knows that their fear is irrational but they also feel as though their conduct is not within their control. The depressed adult knows that their low mood and lack of confidence disables them from carrying out normal family and work obligations expected of them, and this knowledge may fuel their depression further.

See also: *stigma; social exclusion; causes and constructs.*

REFERENCES

Alexander, L.A. and Link, B.G. (2003) 'The impact of contact on stigmatizing attitudes toward people with mental illness', *Journal of Mental Health*, 12 (3): 271–90.

Farina, A. and Felner, R.D. (1973) 'Employment interview reactions to former mental patients', *Journal of Abnormal Psychology*, 82: 268–72.

Garfinkel, H. (1956) 'Conditions of successful degradation ceremonies', *American Journal of Sociology*, 61: 420–4.

Goffman, E. (1961) *Asylums*. Harmondsworth: Penguin.

Gove, W. (1975) 'The labeling theory of mental illness: a reply to Scheff', *American Sociological Review*, 40: 242–8.

Harris, M.J.R., Millich, E.M. and Johnson, D.W. (1990) 'Effects of expectancies on children's social interactions', *Journal of Experimental Social Psychology*, 26: 1–12.

Horwitz, A.V. (1982) *The Social Control of Mental Illness*. New York: Academic Press.
Jones, L. and Cochrane, R. (1981) 'Stereotypes of mental illness: a test of the labelling hypothesis', *International Journal of Social Psychiatry*, 27: 99–107.
Link, B.G. and Phelan, J.C. (1999) 'The labeling theory of mental disorder (II): the consequences of labeling', in A.V. Horwitz and T.L. Scheid (eds), *A Handbook for the Study of Mental Health*. Cambridge: Cambridge University Press.
Rosenhan, D.L. (1973) 'On being sane in insane places', *Science*, 179: 250–8.
Scheff, T. (1966) *Being Mentally Ill: a Sociological Theory*. Chicago: Aldine.
Skinner, L.J., Berry, K.K., Griffiths, S.E. and Byers, B. (1995) 'Generalizability and specificity of the stigma associated with the mental illness label: a reconsideration twenty five years later', *Journal of Community Psychology*, 23: 3–17.
Thoits, P. (1985) 'Self labeling processes in mental illness: the role of emotional deviance', *American Journal of Sociology*, 91: 221–49.
Yarrow, M.J., Schwartz, C., Murphy, H. and Deasy, L. (1955) 'The psychological meaning of mental illness', *Journal of Social Issues*, 11: 12–24.

Stigma

***Definition:* Stigma refers to the social consequences of negative attributions about a person based upon a stereotype. In the case of people with mental health problems, it is presumed that they lack intelligibility and social competence and that they are dangerous.**

Key points: *• The features of stereotyping and stigma are outlined • The particular ways in which people with mental health problems are stereotyped and stigmatized are discussed.*

Stigmatization has two main aspects. First, the person stigmatized is perceived stereotypically as an example of a social group (rather than tentatively and respectfully as an individual). Second, this stereotyping or 'social typing' has negative connotations. (It happens occasionally that there is *positive* stereotyping. This does not lead to stigma but it is still illogical.) These two features are associated with emotional reactions in others such as fear, contempt and disgust, though pity and concern may also be evoked. In the case of the stereotyping of people with mental health problems, all of these reactions may be present in different proportions from one situation to another. Thus stereotyping has both cognitive and emotional aspects.

What then arises from these inner processes of stereotyping is a social reaction, whereby one party rejects that other or reacts towards them in a way that is significantly different. As a result, the stigmatized person is set apart and they suffer the consequences of the social distance created. The person feels depersonalized, rejected and disempowered. As a consequence, they may develop, what Goffman (1963) called a 'spoiled identity'. Pilgrim and Rogers (2005) note that people with mental health problems are stigmatized in a particular way, which refer to three presumed qualities in the target: a lack of intelligibility, a lack of social competence and the presence of violence. The strongest cultural stereotype is the spectre of a homicidal madman – a deranged being who explodes violently, erratically and inexplicably (Foucault, 1978).

In order to establish that stereotyping is irrational, it is necessary to examine the evidence that may or may not support it. In our case here, do mentally ill people always lack intelligibility? Are they always socially incompetent? Are they always violent?

- *The question of intelligibility* In most social situations participants have an obligation, if called upon, to render their speech and conduct intelligible, about any rule transgression or role failure (Goffman, 1971). If we break a rule then we should be able, if called upon, to give an account. If asked, we must be able and willing to provide a persuasive reason or an explanation (Scott and Lyman, 1968). If we do not, then that itself represents a form of rule breaking. With specific regard to madness then this rule breaking does indeed occur. Lay judgements about the emergence of madness refer primarily to the person's lack of intelligibility and inability to explain their oddity in an acceptable or persuasive manner (Coulter, 1973). Of critical importance here is that judgements about the social obligation to explain oneself occur in context. Take the example of talking to oneself. Generally this might be the main piece of behavioural evidence that a person is mad. However, if it happens in church or when the person is holding a mobile telephone to their ear then madness is much less likely to be attributed. Also, the presence of auditory hallucinations may be considered intelligible in one context but not another (these and other points related to the social consequences of stigma are discussed in the sections on Labelling Theory and Madness).

Thus, there *is* some empirical evidence to suggest that the stereotype of people with mental health problems lacking intelligibility is valid. Generally, it is fair to say that mad people act in a way that others do not understand and that they are unable or unwilling to give credible accounts to others of their thoughts and actions. However, there is also evidence that this generalization (the key to stereotyping) is flawed. First, mad people may be unintelligible sometimes and not others. For example it is common for psychosis to occur episodically, with periods of recovery and sanity. Another example is in relation to persistent paranoid delusions. In this case, the person may act completely intelligibly all of the time *except* when the delusional material emerges in conversation. Second, many people with mental health problems (those with a diagnosis of neurosis rather than psychosis) are highly aware of their problems – indeed they may be preoccupied with giving accounts to others about their feelings and actions. The attribution about unintelligibility only applies to madness not all mental disorder and, even then, not all of the time;

- *The question of social competence* Lay judgements about mental health problems and their formal medical codification in psychiatric diagnoses, include an attribution of failed social competence. The mad person loses their credibility because they have lost their reason. Because they are not taken seriously they are socially disabled – they are not permitted to be competent. The depressed or anxious person is unable to carry out their normal role obligations. As with the previous point about intelligibility, there is evidence to undermine these generalizations about the loss of competence (and its associated credibility). First, some people with mental health problems are disproportionately creative. Second, some symptoms create greater competence at some tasks. For example, those with a diagnosis of obsessive-compulsive disorder or obsessive-compulsive personality disorder are more likely to perform above average on tasks requiring a close attention to detail. Third, religious leaders may enjoy heightened credibility, even though they may manifest symptoms of mental illness.

Thus, there is some evidence that some people with mental health problems act in an unintelligible way some of the time. There is no evidence that all people with mental health problems are unintelligible all of the time. Likewise, there is some evidence that some people with mental health problems have diminished social competence, some of the time, to warrant diminished social credibility. However, this is not true all of the time for all people with mental health problems. Indeed, some of the time their competence and credibility is actually raised not diminished. Third, some patients are at increased risk of being violent to others. However, these are in the minority. The great majority of people with a psychiatric diagnosis are not more violent than those without a diagnosis. In some cases, for example in anxious people or in psychotic patients with 'negative symptoms', the probability of violence is actually lower than in the general population.

The persistence of these three elements of stigmatization of those with mental health problems is historically rooted in generalizations made about madness. Not only were these historically based stereotypes always questionable on empirical grounds, they are now applied inappropriately and unfairly to many patients who are not mad. This is because the jurisdiction of contemporary mental health services extends beyond the management of madness. Solutions offered to reverse stigmatization include patients demanding citizenship rights and professionals pleading for mental illness to be treated with the same respect as physical illness. These points are explored further in the section on social exclusion.

See also: *creativity; labelling theory; social exclusion; madness; mental health.*

REFERENCES

Coulter, J. (1973) *Approaches to Insanity*. New York: Wiley.

Foucault, M. (1978) 'About the concept of the "dangerous individual" in 19th century legal psychiatry', *International Journal of Law and Psychiatry*, 1: 1–18.

Goffman, E. (1963) *Stigma: Some Notes on the Management of Spoiled Identity*. Harmondsworth: Penguin.

Goffman, E. (1971) *Relations in Public*. Harmondsworth: Penguin.

Pilgrim, D. and Rogers, A. (2005) *A Sociology of Mental Health and Illness (Third Edition)*. Maidenhead: Open University Press.

Scott, M.B. and Lyman, S.M. (1968) 'Accounts', *American Journal of Sociology*, 33.

Social Exclusion

Definition: Social exclusion refers to the various ways in which an individual or group of individuals are denied access to levels of citizenship, social association and wealth available to others.

Key points: • *Examples are given of the social exclusion of people with mental health problems • A focus on social exclusion is contrasted with the traditional emphasis on stigma.*

A number of entries in this book emphasize the negative social consequences of receiving a psychiatric diagnosis and having service contact. While the causes of mental health problems may remain contested, their consequences (whether viewed as direct impairment or constructed disability) are very clear. Those with mental health problems experience social exclusion on a number of fronts:

- *Labour market disadvantage* Psychiatric patients are often unemployed and their history may jeopardize any future employment. Only a minority of psychotic patients will find work (Jenkins and Singh, 2001). Neurotic patients are four times more likely to be unemployed than non-patients and five times more likely to be receiving invalidity benefits than the general population (Rogers and Pilgrim, 2003). People with mental health problems are nearly three times as likely as physically disabled people of being unemployed (Department for Education and Employment, 1998). Chronic unemployment feeds demoralization and, in the case of psychotic patients, increases their chances of relapse (Warner, 1985);
- *Derision and hostility from the mass media* The mass media both reflect and encourage public hostility and distrust towards people with mental health problems. In particular newspapers are disproportionately prone to publish stories which link mental health problems to violence (Philo et al., 1994). By contrast little is said about patients as victims of violence or as productive or creative

members of society. The norms about discriminatory reporting are evident in headlines such as 'Schizophrenic kills . . .' (newspapers would not print 'Black kills . . .'). Also the mass media will use ordinary language descriptions of madness in a silly humorous way in stories ('Looney council . . .'). This tendency to make mental health a source of either anxiety or trivial humour creates the conditions under which media audiences are more likely to reject and distrust people with mental health problems;

- *Poverty* This is wider than labour market disadvantage but in part flows from it. People with mental health problems are more likely to live in socially disorganized and poor localities. In the latter are high levels of noise, pollution, litter and traffic congestion. In addition to these environmental stressors, social networks are weak and crime rates high. Those with mental health problems who remain chronically unemployed have to suffer the shared consequences with others in this situation. Daily life is unstructured and meaningful activity may be unavailable. The comforts of substance misuse may fill the void this desolate culture creates. Substance misuse amplifies mental health problems and undermines physical health. Poverty means that stress-reduction activities (such as holidays) are restricted. Thus a whole range of cultural and economic processes impinge on poor people. Those with pre-existing mental health problems are particularly vulnerable to these negative social forces;
- *Lawful discrimination* People who have inpatient stays in acute mental health services are detained in unusual circumstances. Typically, they will have committed no crime. No one will have acted as an advocate to argue against their admission – all of the professional procedures are aimed at formalizing a consensus for the decision. Although they may be recorded, officially, as being a 'voluntary' or 'informal' patient, they may have been given no genuine choice. It is common for patients to enter hospital in a pseudo-voluntary state. They are told that if they do not 'come quietly' then powers of involuntary detention will be invoked (Rogers, 1993). If they resist detention or seek to leave hospital, then staff members are provided with legal powers to physically restrain them. If they refuse medication it may be imposed upon them. They may be isolated in a room ('secluded'). While there are safeguards against excesses and misuse in these regards, there is clear daily empirical evidence that a psychiatric diagnosis brings with it a range of risks to any patient's privacy and autonomy. Together, these legal powers also create

> particular ways in which people with mental health problems are excluded from society. Once limited to hospitals, they are now being extended increasingly to community settings (Dennis and Monahan, 1996).

It is clear then that, on a number of fronts, people with mental health problems are socially excluded. Evidence about this broader set of social forces constraining the welfare and citizenship of patients has led some commentators to criticize the stigma framework. For example Sayce (2000) argues that the latter reduces the field of inquiry to that of the characteristics and plight of stigmatized *individuals*. Sayce argues that we should instead examine the *collective* discriminatory response of others. The four areas of discrimination noted above together provide this collective response.

Sayce points out that although the frame of individual stereotyping needs to be widened to look at collective responses, the cognitive features of the latter are still an important starting point to understand a range of stances in society, about the social inclusion or exclusion of people with mental health problems. She notes that different interest groups manifest different assumptions about three inter-related aspects of discrimination towards people with mental health problems: the nature of mental health problems; the causes of mental health problems; what should be done about discrimination.

If a psychiatrist or the relative of a patient considers that the latter is suffering from a genetically caused disturbance of brain biochemistry, then they will argue that discrimination will be reduced by campaigning for us all to accept mental illness to be like any other illness. Moreover, they would also demand more research into the (putative) genetic causes of mental illness, now framed as a brain disease, in order to reduce the prevalence of future 'sufferers'. The latter term is common within this approach because patients are seen as diseased victims of biological misfortune (being born with the wrong genes). By contrast, a service user who argues that psychological difference is caused by a variety of oppressive factors will argue for social change and the right to full citizenship and so the reduction or abolition of compulsory psychiatric treatment.

Take another example. A biological view of depression might lead to an educational campaign to encourage patients to seek anti-depressant treatment. For this reason the drug companies in their marketing strategies depict depression in a matter of fact way as a biological illness. Social inclusion in this context would be limited to an equal right to medical treatment. By contrast an environmental etiological view would lead to calls for reductions in social stressors (like poverty, work stress and so on) (Goldstein and Rosselli, 2003). Social inclusion in this context would be about people with mental health problems having access to benign and supportive living environments and to satisfying work roles.

The representations of different diagnostic groups by others can also affect degrees of treatment equity within mental health services. For example, mental health workers tend to be paternalistic towards psychotic patients but distrusting and rejecting towards those with a diagnosis of personality disorder (Markham, 2003). Both are stigmatized groups but different attributions about personal 'fault' from professionals lead to differential levels of personal acceptance and support.

See also: *stigma; labelling theory; the mental health service users' movement; social class.*

REFERENCES

Dennis, D.L. and Monahan, J. (eds) (1996) *Coercion and Aggressive Community Treatment*. New York: Plenum Press.

Department for Education and Employment (DfEE) (1998) *Labour Force Survey: Unemployment and Activity Rates for People of Working Age*. London: DfEE.

Goldstein, B. and Rosselli, F. (2003) 'Etiological paradigms of depression: the relationship between perceived causes, empowerment, treatment preferences and stigma', *Journal of Mental Health*, 12 (4): 551–64.

Jenkins, R. and Singh, B. (2001) 'Mental disorder and disability in the population', in G. Thornicroft and G. Szmuckler (eds), *Textbook of Community Psychiatry*. Oxford: Oxford University Press.

Markham, D. (2003) 'Attitudes towards patients with a diagnosis of "borderline personality disorder": social rejection and dangerousness', *Journal of Mental Health* 12, (6): 595–612.

Philo, G., Secker, J., Platt, S., Henderson, L., McLaughlin, G. and Burnside, J. (1994) 'The impact of the mass media on public images of mental illness', *Health Education Journal*, 53: 271–81.

Rogers, A. (1993) 'Coercion and voluntary admissions: an examination of psychiatric patients' views', *Behavioural Sciences and the Law*, 11: 259–68.

Rogers, A. and Pilgrim, D. (2003) *Inequality and Mental Health*. Basingstoke: Palgrave.

Sayce, L. (2000) *From Psychiatric Patient to Citizen: Overcoming Discrimination and Social Exclusion*. Basingstoke: Macmillan.

Warner, R. (1985) *Recovery from Schizophrenia: Psychiatry and Political Economy*. London: Routledge.

Risks to and from People with Mental Health Problems

Definition: People with mental health problems may be a source of risk to themselves and others. They are also subject to particular risks from others and their environment.

Key points: *• The evidence for and against the stereotype that psychiatric patients are dangerous is reviewed • The evidence about psychiatric patients being at risk from others is reviewed.*

The dominant cultural image of mental disorder (dating back to antiquity) is one of violence. The problem with this dominant image is that it is stereotypical. It is empirically inaccurate and, for the majority of people with mental health problems, it is a source of unfair treatment (in its widest sense).

In order to bring both accuracy and justice into the debates about mental health problems and dangerousness a number of points can be made:

- *Because the concept of mental disorder is now very wide, it includes some highly dangerous people* The continued association between violence and psychiatric diagnosis now does have some empirical basis. The reason for this is that two broad diagnostic groups (those who abuse substances and those with a diagnosis of anti-social personality disorder) have significantly high rates of violence. Indeed, in the case of anti-social personality disorder, violence (sexual or otherwise) is central to its circular definition. As psychiatry developed in the twentieth century its jurisdiction extended from lunacy to include personality disorder and substance misuse. This now means that people with these diagnoses are psychiatric patients and so encourage and maintain the stereotype that *all* psychiatric patients are dangerous (Pilgrim and Rogers, 2003);

- *Substance abuse and personality disorder, not psychosis, are the best predictors of violence* The above point begs a question: are people with a diagnosis other than substance misuse or anti-social personality disorder prone to violence? The answer is 'no'. Indeed most psychotic and the overwhelming majority of neurotic patients are no more violent than the general population (Steadman et al., 1998). This point is also true of many forms of personality disorder. There is an important exception to this trend: those with 'co-morbidity' or 'dual diagnosis'. Psychotic patients who abuse substances are significantly more violent than either the general population or psychotic patients who do not abuse substances. Similarly, some mentally disordered offenders are given a dual diagnosis of mental illness and personality disorder. Substance misuse and anti-social personality disorder are highly predictive of violence to others. Psychotic patients with positive symptoms (hallucinations and delusions) who abuse substances are significantly more dangerous (Soyka, 2000). Thus the key issue here is that psychosis alone is not an indicator of risk to others, despite the long-standing stereotype implying such a relationship. It is the co-presence of substance abuse and/or personality problems that raises the probability of violence in psychiatric populations. This co-presence is important for another reason: psychiatric patients live in circumstances in which the comforts of substance abuse are common. They are three to four times more likely to abuse substances than the general population (Regier et al., 1990). Between 20% and 30% of psychotic patients living in the community are likely to abuse substances (Hambracht and Hafner, 1996);
- *Iatrogenic damage and loss of liberty* The largest risk to patients is from service contact. Most admissions to acute units are now involuntary, so patients are at a high risk of losing their liberty without trial. Also all forms of treatment, both biological and psychological, carry risks (see the sections on these two). Apart from the risk created by professional action, patients are also at risk of stigma from service contact. Hospitalization also disrupts community living and may even jeapordize tenancy arrangements;
- *Crime* Because psychiatric patients are often poor, they tend to live in poor community contexts with higher crime rates. For this reason patients run a high risk of being victims of both acquisitive and violent

crime. They are also at risk of becoming criminals because of local cultural norms. Patients typically live in what Silver and colleagues (1999) call 'concentrated poverty'. These living conditions contain more 'violence-inducing social forces' which impact upon patients as potential victims and perpetrators (Hiday, 1995). For this reason discussions about patients in either role need to take into account ecological factors not just the clinical and personality characteristics of individuals (Rogers and Pilgrim, 2003);

- *Risks associated with poverty* In addition to the risk of being victims of crime, poor living circumstances also bring with them peculiar stressors: congested traffic, litter, air pollution, poorer access to health care and education and fewer leisure facilities. They also mean that stress-reducing options (such as vacations) are reduced;
- *Suicide* This is discussed in a separate entry. Here it will simply be noted that people with mental health problems live shorter lives than others. Most of this loss of years alive is as a result of suicide;
- *'The manner in which one is dangerous'* This phrase was used by Szasz (1963) to make the point that psychiatric patients suffer discrimination. Some dangerous roles are highly rewarded and bring with them raised social status (e.g. boxers, mountaineers, racing drivers and astronauts). Also some forms of injurious and self-injurious behaviour does not lead to the actors being readily detained without trial (smoking, fast driving). Moreover, the rules of detention about dangerousness are applied differently to patients. They may lose their liberty without trial for *predicted future action*. By contrast, other violent citizens only risk loss of liberty as a consequence of *proven past action*. The due process of a court trial allows the accused to argue for their innocence and freedom and they are provided with an advocate to support these arguments. By contrast, the civil detention of psychiatric patients occurs without court proceedings and the patient is not provided with the opportunity to argue for their continued liberty with the support of a legal advocate.

To conclude, any comprehensive discussion of the issue of risk and mental health problems has to consider a two-way process. While media reports and public prejudice may focus disproportionately on one aspect (violent risk to others), the reality is that it is risks to patients which are more prevalent – ones of iatrogenic damage, poverty and premature death. Moreover, patients enjoy less legal protection than others when their risk to others is being investigated and dealt with.

See also: *suicide; biological interventions; psychological interventions; the mass media; stigma.*

REFERENCES

Hambracht, M. and Hafner, H. (1996) 'Substance abuse and the onset of schizophrenia', *Biological Psychiatry*, 40: 1155–63.

Hiday, V. (1995) 'The social context of mental illness and violence', *Journal of Health and Social Behaviour*, 36: 122–37.

Pilgrim, D. and Rogers, A. (2003) 'Mental disorder and violence: an empirical picture in context', *Journal of Mental Health*, 12 (1): 7–18.

Regier, D.A., Farmer, M.E., Rae, D.S., Locke, B.J., Keith, S.J., Judd, L.L. and Goddwin, F.K. (1990) 'Comorbidity of mental disorders with alcohol and other drug use: results from the epidemiologic catchment area (ECA) study', *Journal of the American Medical Association*, 264: 2511–18.

Rogers, A. and Pilgrim, D. (2003) *Mental Health and Inequality*. Basingstoke: Palgrave.

Silver, E., Mulvey, E.P. and Monahan, J. (1999) 'Assessing violence risk among discharged psychiatric patients: towards an ecological approach', *Law and Human Behavior*, 23: 237–55.

Soyka, M. (2000) 'Substance misuse, psychiatric disorder and violent and disturbed behaviour', *British Journal of Psychiatry*, 176: 345–50.

Steadman, H.J., Mulvey, E.P., Monahan, J., Robbins, P.C., Applebaum, P.S., Grisso, T., Roth, L.H. and Silver, E. (1998) 'Violence by people discharged from acute psychiatric facilities and by others in the same neighbourhood', *Archives of General Psychiatry*, 55: 109.

Szasz, T.S. (1963) *Law, Liberty and Psychiatry*. New York: Macmillan.

The Mass Media

***Definition:* The mass media refer to outlets of information and entertainment, such as radio, television, cinema and newspapers. The role of the mass media in maintaining negative images of people with mental health problems has been the focus of substantial criticism.**

Key points: • *The role of the mass media in reinforcing and maintaining prejudice against people with mental health problems is examined* • *Some recent counter-examples from radio programmes and the cinema are described.*

The definition above refers to 'outlets of information and entertainment'. The blurring of the boundaries between the two is reflected in the notion of 'infotainment' – the tendency of the mass media to maximize audience levels by mixing information with strategies of shock and titillation. The more serious is the intention of the journalist and the ethos of particular outlets within the media, the more likely it is that empirical findings and even-handed analysis are privileged over entertainment. The long-standing stereotypes of mental health problems being linked to violence and derision mean that they are ready-made topics for journalistic interest. People with mental health problems are also vulnerable when distressed and lack credibility because of their defined loss of reason. This makes them easy targets for negative news stories and story lines.

Historically, negative images about madness preceded the emergence of the mass media (Rosen, 1968). For this reason, it is not logical to argue that the latter simply create negative images of mental health problems in modern society. It is relevant though to examine the role played by the mass media in maintaining and amplifying such images and to provide an empirical and ethical critique of this role. The educational role of the mass media about mental health problems is significant. For example, surveys of public opinion about mental illness reveal that the mass media are the main source of information for lay people (Wahl, 1995).

Within media depictions, there is an overwhelming emphasis on violence. This is true of newspaper news stories (e.g. Angermeyer and Schulze, 2001) as well as TV fictional portrayals (e.g. Signorielli, 1989). This trend seems to be consistent and global for the various countries studied: USA (Diefenbach, 1997); Canada (Day and Page, 1986); Germany (Angermeyer and Schulze, 2001); New Zealand (Nairn et al., 2001); and Britain (Philo et al., 1994; Rose, 1998). The trend of violent portrayal may be amplifying, with people with mental health problems being depicted as being even more dangerous than 50 years ago (Phelan et al., 2000). Sieff (2003) points out that while there has been a recent increase in the occurrence of positive images, these tend to be limited to people with anxiety or depressive symptoms. The link between psychosis and violence and unpredictability remains very strong.

Cinematic presentations of mental health problems have tended to reflect and reinforce this stereotype of violence but, recently, more positive or sympathetic images can be found in mainstream film-making (e.g. *A Beautiful Mind*). They can also be found in some films where a minor character has a mental health problem (e.g. *Just a Boy)*.These are a recent corrective to a long tradition of film-making in which mental health problems are associated only with either violence or ridicule.

The mass media have also provided an occasional opportunity for mental health issues to be discussed seriously. For example, two of the public inquiries into the mistreatment of patients in the two English Special Hospitals of Rampton (1980) and Ashworth (1991) were triggered by investigative TV programmes.

An earlier example was the interest taken by the *That's Life* programme in the 1970s about tranquillizer use. It is noteworthy that this began as a collaborative campaign with MIND (the National Association of Mental Health) about the problems of anti-psychotic medication (*major* tranquillizers). However, the programme was deluged with interest from the watching public about addiction to benzodiazepines (*minor* tranquillizers). This indicates that the role of the mass media has to be understood as an interaction with its recipient audiences rather than as a one-way source of influence. It also reflects the power differential between the two medicated groups, with psychotic patients being displaced by neurotic patients.

Other examples of serious consideration about mental health matters in the mass media in recent years have been programmes such as *All in the Mind* and *In the Psychiatrist's Chair* on the BBC's Radio Four. These allow professionals and patients to offer a voice to the general public and discuss research about mental health issues. They are not sensationalist nor do they contribute to scaremongering and public prejudice. Indeed, it is the newspapers (especially but not uniquely the tabloids) which are most prone to these negative interventions.

See also: *stigma; labelling theory; social exclusion.*

REFERENCES

Angermeyer, M.C. and Schulze, B. (2001) 'Reinforcing stereotypes: how the focus on forensic cases in news reporting may influence public attitudes towards the mentally ill', *International Journal of Law and Psychiatry*, 24: 469–86.

Day, D.M. and Page, S. (1986) 'Portrayal of mental illness in Canadian newspapers', *Canadian Journal of Psychiatry*, 31: 813–17.

Diefenbach, D. (1997) 'The portrayal of mental illness on prime-time television', *Journal of Community Psychology*, 43 (4): 51–8.

Nairn, R., Coverdale, J. and Claasen, D. (2001) 'From source material to news story in New Zealand print media: a prospective study of the stigmatizing processes in depicting mental illness', *Australian and New Zealand Journal of Psychiatry*, 35 (5): 654–9.

Phelan, J.C., Link, B.G., Stueve, A. and Pescosolido, B.A. (2000) 'Public conceptions of mental illness in 1950 and 1996: what is mental illness and is it to be feared?', *Journal of Health and Social Behaviour*, 41: 188–207.

Philo, G., Secker, J., Platt, S., Henderson, L., McLaughlin, G. and Burnside, J. (1994) 'The

impact of the mass media on public images of mental illness: media content and audience belief', *Health Education Journal*, 53: 271–81.
Rose, D. (1998) 'Television madness and community care', *Journal of Applied Community Social Psychology*, 8: 213–28.
Rosen, G. (1968) *Madness in Society*. New York: Harper.
Sieff, E.M. (2003) 'Media frames of mental illnesses: the potential impact of negative frames', *Journal of Mental Health*, 12 (3): 259–69.
Signorielli, N. (1989) 'The stigma of mental illness on television', *Journal of Broadcasting and Electronic Media*, 33 (3): 325–31.
Wahl, O.F. (1995) *Media Madness: Public Images of Mental Illness*. New York: Rutgers University Press.

Suicide

***Definition:* Deliberate, self-imposed death.**

Key points: *• The error of conflating suicide with mental disorder is noted • A range of points are summarized about the complexity of the topic.*

A paradox of this entry is that it contributes further to a criticism about to be made – that suicide is seen, all too readily and singularly, as a mental health problem. The entry makes a small further contribution to this fundamental error of reasoning but, in its defence, it will also try to correct the error. Suicide is a complex topic and will be discussed here under a number of points:

- *Suicide is a crude and at times misleading proxy for mental health* There are a number of problems with any policy measure which conflates suicide and mental disorder. Suicide is not necessarily irrational. There are many circumstances in which a resolution of personal suffering is for the individual to make a logical decision to end his or her life. Also, in some cultures or circumstances suicide has been seen as an honourable, not a dysfunctional, act. For example, the traditional Japanese phenomena of *hara-kiri* and *kamikaze* indicate that death at one's own hands can be both appropriate and honourable (and certainly not a symptom of psychopathology). Another example of this question of rationality and honour is in relation to *jauhar*. This was a ritual of collective female suicide in Hindus in medieval India, when faced with invading Muslim hordes. Death was a preferred option to degradation and slavery.

More ambiguously, some religious cults have attracted attention, when their leaders have demanded obedience about mass suicide (e.g. the Waco suicides in Texas and the Heaven's Gate suicides in California). The ambiguity surrounds value judgements about cults. Are they an example of mass mental disorder? Are their leaders grandiose and sadistic and their followers dependent and masochistic? Did all of the current accepted major world religions start as small cults?

The main point here is that there is a danger of irrationality being imputed retrospectively in all cases. That is, when and if a person commits suicide then it is easy to argue that the 'balance of their mind' was faulty at the fatal moment or that they had a prior mental disorder, which made them particularly prone to self-sacrifice. Such a conclusion is by no means always logically warranted. Moreover, in older people with multiple physical illness there may be an understandable wish to die. This can lead to the *post hoc* psychiatric attribution of mental illness (depression) in this group, which is deemed to warrant treatment. This is not to say that suicide some of the time may well reflect irrational reasoning. What cannot be legitimately claimed, though, is that suicide *always and necessarily* reflects irrationality;

- *There are international and intra-national differences in suicide profiles* Differences occur in the preferred type of suicide and the rate of suicide. In the USA guns are the preferred option (reflecting their availability). By contrast in relatively gun-free cultures like in Britain, carbon monoxide poisoning from car exhaust fumes is the main option used by men (women are more likely to use pills to self-poison). Suicide rates are at their highest in Northern, Central and Eastern Europe (including Russia) and North America. They are at their lowest in the Mediterranean and Islamic countries. These patterns may change over time. For example, Durkheim (1951) in his classic sociological study of suicide noted that during wartime the suicide rate drops. It increases during peaks in both prosperity and relative poverty. More recent evidence suggests that areas with high rates of poverty, poor employment, unemployment and poor local social cohesion witness higher suicide rates. There are also occupational differences, with medical practitioners and farmers being at a higher risk than the general population;

- *There are age and gender differences in suicidal behaviour* Across the life span, there is a global pattern of men completing suicide more frequently than women. However, attempted suicide is more common in young women than young men (a ratio of about 2:1). For emphasis, though, it can be noted that more young men commit suicide than do women. The tendency for attempted suicide to peak in younger years may reflect the relative powerlessness of the young, with a suicidal gesture being powerful;
- *Some, but not all, self-harming reflects suicidal behaviour* Many people who self-harm (for example when cutting themselves) are very clear that they are not suicidal. Some self-harm activity is mainly directed at tension release or self-punishment – it does not signal a wish to die. Moreover, in some people dramatic suicidal gestures are used as a communication to influence others (as in the actions of histrionic personalities when they are distressed). In the psychiatric literature suicide (or 'completed' suicide) is usually distinguished from suicide attempts or 'parasuicide'. There are both empirical and cultural problems with this distinction. For example, a person who is found dying at their own hands may or may not be relieved if they are saved by others. An alternative example is that a person may not intend to commit suicide in a dramatic gesture which 'goes wrong'.

  In cultures where there is a shame attached to suicide (or where it is illegal) parasuicide may be under-reported. For example in India suicidal behaviour is still a punishable legal offence. Suicide is also considered to be immoral according to some forms of strict religious observance. The moral and legal context can thus shape norms of reporting about suicidal behaviour. A final empirical problem is that an open verdict is often recorded of people dying at their own hands, this makes precise estimates of suicide difficult and brings into question the validity of suicide data at times;
- *People with mental health problems are at greater risk of suicide* The reasons for this are contested and can be related back to the basic cultural assumption addressed at the outset (that suicidal action is always irrational). Empirically the picture is by no means clear. For example, depressed behaviour seems to be linked to a tendency to commit suicide. However, not all depressed people commit suicide and some who show no obvious symptoms of depression can

(shockingly) take their own life. Despite seasonal variations in mood (particularly in Northern Europe) suicide rates do not increase in the winter but are at their highest in the spring and summer. Women receive a psychiatric diagnosis more often than men but the latter commit suicide more often than the former. Having said all of this, some mental health problems are associated with an increased risk of suicide. Depressed patients who are older, male and abuse substances are at a significantly high risk. Those with a diagnosis of schizophrenia are also at a significantly high risk of suicide. Factors which might affect this correlation are loss of career or academic success, social exclusion and the impact of anti-psychotic medication, which includes distressing agitation (akathisia) and a drop in mood (acute dysphoria). Those with a diagnosis of schizophrenia are at a 14-fold rate of risk compared to the general population and in the case of bi-polar disorder it is a 12-fold risk. However, despite these psychiatric correlations and the sociological trends noted above, no successful method has been found to accurately predict risk of an *individual* committing suicide in either clinical or non-clinical populations.

See also: *risks to and from people with mental health problems; physical health; biological interventions.*

FURTHER READING

Durkheim, E. (1951) *Suicide: a Study in Sociology*. Glencoe: Free Press.

Firestone, R.W. (1997) *Suicide and the Inner Voice*. Thousand Oaks, CA: SAGE Publications.

Hawton, K.E. and van Heeringen, K. (2000) *The International Handbook of Suicide and Attempted Suicide*. Chichester: Wiley.

O'Connor, R.C. and Sheehy, N.P. (2001) 'Suicidal behaviour', *The Psychologist*, 14 (1): 20–4.

The Mental Health Service Users' Movement

***Definition:* The mental health service users' movement is an international network of people with mental health problems who are critical of orthodox psychiatric theory and practice and who demand full rights of citizenship.**

Key points: *• Different ways of understanding the role of psychiatric patients are discussed • One of these (the 'survivor') is elaborated in relation to new social movements • The concerns and demands of the mental health service users' movement are described.*

Those studying the accounts of psychiatric patients living in the community have found that they have a number of daily concerns about social exclusion and their ability to cope in poor conditions of support (Barham and Hayward, 1991). Patients who are in contact with specialist mental health services are also critical of the way professionals frame their problems, the use of coercion and the narrow range of treatment responses offered (Rogers et al., 1993).

Rogers and Pilgrim (2005) point out that mental health service users can be thought of in four ways: as patients; as consumers; as survivors; or as providers. Literature about the third use of the term user, 'survivor', emphasizes the collective oppression of psychiatric patients by mental health services and their wider host society. The term 'survivor' is itself ambiguous. It can indicate that a person has survived their mental health problem and it can refer to surviving the ordeal of mental health service contact. The term 'mental health service users' movement' is used here, but it is not universal. In the USA, where the term 'user' strongly connotes substance misuse, the term 'ex-patient' tends to be preferred.

Even in the UK as well as 'users' movement', the term 'survivors' movement' can also be found.

Dutch literature alludes to an 'opposition movement'. The latter is useful because it points up an important bias in the movement. Although they make demands about citizenship, much of the anger and debates of disaffected patients focus on disappointments or frustrations about the psychiatric profession and mental health services. This antagonistic link to psychiatry is exemplified in *Shrink Resistant: the Struggle Against Psychiatry in Canada* by Burstow and Weitz (1988). Given this disaffection about psychiatry and mental health services, the term 'user' is problematic because patients do not always see services as being 'of use', nor is the contact always voluntary. Whether this contact means that they 'use a service' is a moot point. It suggests that third parties, benefiting from the patients' removal from society, might be the real users of services.

The reactions of psychiatry to these attacks have been mixed. Sometimes they are dismissed as the collective and unreliable accounts of people who, by definition have lost their reason (they are mentally ill). At other times, though, the criticisms have been taken seriously, particularly by that group of critical psychiatrists forming the 'post-psychiatry' movement. The focus on the failings of psychiatry also links the mental health service users' movement to 'anti-psychiatry', with the latter being built on and endorsed favourably by movement members.

The mental health service users' movement grew in the 1970s in the USA and mainland Europe, and in the mid-1980s in the UK (Campbell, 1996; Rogers and Pilgrim, 1991). It can be thought of as one example of a new social movement. The latter is a group containing people with a common identity, who seek to promote their interests in opposition to dominant forms of power and organization preferred by the State (Toch, 1965). The obvious examples of this are the women's movement, the black consciousness movement, the disability movement and the ecology movement. These can be distinguished from older social movements, like versions of the labour or workers' movement, which focus on formal bureaucratic forms of organization and on economic and politic demands. By contrast, new social movements are less bureaucratic and they tend to make wider demands about personal liberation and citizenship or, in the case of ecology, the prevention of global disaster. They emphasize civil not just political demands and they establish new agendas outside of the normal democratic processes of the State bureaucracy (Habermas, 1981).

If they can be characterized in traditional political terms at all, the new social movements tend to have a mixture of liberal, left-libertarian and anarchist values. These generalizations need to be tentative though. For example, some parts of the black consciousness movement show marked authoritarian and patriarchal tendencies. Sometimes the term 'identity politics' is also used to capture the nature of new social movements. However, the ecology movement does not neatly fit this definition.

Turning to the content of the mental health service users' movement, a number of themes can be identified:

- *The opposition to coercion* The focus here is on the way in which mental health problems are segregated forcibly from society;
- *The opposition to compulsory treatment* As well as the issue of compulsory detention, compulsory treatment is also opposed. Indeed the notion of medical treatment is inherently problematic if it is imposed. Assaults on resistant bodies are cast as 'treatment' because the State delegates lawful powers to professionals. Similarly what is solitary confinement in prison becomes 'seclusion' in mental health services. The users' movement seeks to expose the mystification of these oppressive practices carried out under the cloak of medical paternalism;
- *The opposition to psychiatric diagnosis* This varies in its salience in the movement but many patients resent the application of a medical diagnosis to a problem they prefer to frame in biographical, social or spiritual terms;
- *The demand for greater treatment choice* This relates to the dominant use of physical treatments in psychiatry. Users demand a greater choice of treatment responses than are on offer. Common demands are for psychosurgery and electroconvulsive therapy to be outlawed and for psychological therapies to be more available;
- *The demand for greater citizenship* This feature is shared with the physical disability movement. It is the one area of demand that lies outside complaints about psychiatry and specialist services, though the latter may still be criticized for not promoting social inclusion.

Earlier the notion of user-as-consumer was noted. This has had the effect of diverting time and energy from the new social movement of psychiatric patients. The consumer emphasis is associated with 'user involvement' in mental health services (Pilgrim and Waldron, 1998). This draws users into the narrower agenda of the State's reforms of its pre-existing forms of organization; professionally dominated mental health services.

See also: *'anti-psychiatry'; the 'myth of mental illness'; mental health; service-user involvement.*

REFERENCES

Barham, P. and Hayward, R. (1991) *From the Mental Patient to the Person.* London: Routledge.

Burstow, B. and Weitz, D. (eds) (1988) *Shrink Resistant: the Struggle Against Psychiatry in Canada.* Vancouver: New Star.

Campbell, P. (1996) 'The history of the user movement in the United Kingdom', in T. Heller, J. Reynolds, R. Gomm, R. Muston and S. Pattison (eds), *Mental Health Matters.* Basingstoke: Macmillan.

Habermas, J. (1981) 'New social movements', *Telos*, 48:33–7.

Pilgrim, D. and Waldron, L. (1998) 'User involvement in mental health service development: how far can it go?', *Journal of Mental Health*, 7 (1): 95–104.

Rogers, A. and Pilgrim, D. (1991) '"Pulling down churches": accounting for the mental health users' movement', *Sociology of Health and Illness*, 13 (2): 129–48.

Rogers, A. and Pilgrim, D. (2005) *A Sociology of Mental Health and Illness (Third Edition).* Maidenhead: Open University Press.

Rogers, A., Pilgrim, D. and Lacey, R. (1993) *Experiencing Psychiatry: Users' Views of Services.* Basingstoke: MIND/Macmillan.

Toch, H. (1965) *The Social Psychology of Social Movements.* New York: Bobbs Merrill.

Cross-cultural Psychiatry

***Definition:* This refers to the branch of psychiatry which compares and contrasts manifestations of mental disorder in different cultures.**

Key points: *• Cross-cultural psychiatry is outlined • Two readings of cross-cultural psychiatry are given, one orthodox and the other sceptical.*

Cross-cultural (or 'transcultural') psychiatry can be explored in two ways. It can simply be read as a source of knowledge about mental disorder in different cultures. Alternatively, the contradictions it exposes about psychiatric knowledge are also noteworthy. In the first, a universal body of psychiatric knowledge is considered to be non-problematic. The main interest is then in the study of differences *within* this assumed universally legitimate body of knowledge. In the second, psychiatric knowledge is read sceptically, and cross cultural differences are deemed to expose further the futility of claims of a unifying and valid body of psychiatric knowledge. This entry will consider both readings.

CULTURAL DIFFERENCES IN MENTAL DISORDER – THE ORTHODOX READING

Cross-cultural psychiatry starts with three assumptions. First, it is assumed that mental disorder, as defined and studied by Western psychiatry (developed in the nineteenth century mainly from German psychiatric diagnosis and classification – 'nosology'), is manifested universally. It is taken as read that the definitions of mental disorder set out by *DSM* and *ICD* (see the section on Psychiatric Diagnosis) are valid. Thus, say 'depression' or 'schizophrenia' are considered to be valid diagnoses, with stable symptom profiles, that can be investigated internationally. The second assumption is that specific forms of mental disorder may be shaped in their expression, incidence and prevalence by cultural differences. An implication of this is that psychiatrists should be very careful to understand cultural meanings (especially semantic subtleties, non-verbal etiquette and folk belief systems) when making any diagnosis. Third, there is an assumption that sometimes there are expressions of mental abnormality which are culturally unique.

It is in this third area that cross-cultural psychiatry attracts most attention in Western readers because of the exotic connotations of what are called 'culturally related specific syndromes'. For example, in Malaya some men have a morbid fear that their penis is shrinking and that this is an indication of imminent death (*koro*). A female version of this is in relation to shrinking nipples. A similar genital fear is found in India, called the *dhat* syndrome. This is the belief that serious illness will be created by excessive loss of sperm (from nocturnal emission or masturbation). In another example, in China there is a morbid fear of catching colds (frigophobia; *pa-len*; *wei-han*). This is in the context of the Chinese belief system about the balance between yin and yang. Those with a fear of colds predominating will over-dress in warm weather and avoid cold-inducing foods.

In Japan, with its particular sensitivity to the views of others, some adolescents develop *taijinkyofushio*. This entails the young person being excessively anxious about how they are viewed by others, especially classmates and others they must socially encounter, who are not family members. A final example is Nigerian brain fag syndrome. This is the anxious belief on the part of the patient that their intellectual and sensory capacities are impaired, accompanied by a burning sensation in the head and neck.

CULTURAL DIFFERENCES IN MENTAL DISORDER – THE SCEPTICAL READING

The central problem for cross-cultural psychiatry is that if it introduces too much sensitivity to cultural differences (a form of relativism) then the core assumption about a universally stable body of knowledge is under threat. If, on the other hand, the latter is over-emphasized then psychiatrists are accused of being culturally insensitive or of manifesting a form of Western cultural imperialism. The use of American society as a normative cultural base for *DSM* encourages this criticism. Those committed to cross-cultural psychiatry can either be accused of 'having it both ways', in their attitude towards the universal and the particular, or they are constantly struggling to advocate the correct or delicate balance between them.

In support of the universal hypothesis is that some conditioned physiological processes (anxiety and the misery linked to 'learned helplessness') are demonstrably universal (see the sections on Sadness and Fear). Moreover, some broad generalizations can be made about these phenomena in other mammals, not just about all human beings. The problem comes when these expressions of distress are reified or codified using Western medical labels. Why should Western labels (specifically nineteenth-century Germanic ones) be deemed to be intrinsically valid or superior to ones preferred elsewhere? Also why are these labels medical in nature? Why are medical codifications superior to religious or social ones or ordinary language descriptions?

These questions arise because of the centrality of language in human functioning. This allows us to rehearse alternative meanings for what we experience and what we see. This open textured reflectiveness allows us, for example, to view anxiety in ourselves or others as an illness or as an existential state (or both). Depression can be viewed as an illness or experienced as a religious experience invoked by sin. Why is the first right and the second wrong? Who decides? When it comes to madness (see the entry with that name) why is it mental illness rather than unrecognized creativity, religious insight or simply a mystery to be tolerated? These questions undermine our confidence in the universal applicability of psychiatric knowledge.

Despite these criticisms invited by cross-cultural psychiatry, the latter provides an opportunity to discuss cultural relativism. It also encourages orthodox Western practitioners to be more sensitive to alternative belief systems and contextual reasoning. In doing so, it invites them to pay close attention to the particular meanings being expressed by an individual patient. Genuine cross-cultural sensitivity may ensure that psychiatrists provide unique formulations when they encounter patients from alien cultures. Ironically, this habit is not encouraged by the application of standard diagnostic techniques, based upon *DSM* or *ICD*, within a Western native culture.

See also: *race; psychiatric diagnosis; fear; sadness; madness.*

FURTHER READING

Abas, M., Broadhead, J.C., Mbape, P. and Khumalo-Satakukwa, G. (1994) 'Defeating depression in the developing world', *British Journal of Psychiatry*, 164: 293–6.

Kleinman, A. (1988) *Rethinking Psychiatry*. New York: Free Press.

Tseng, W-S. (2003) *Clinician's Guide to Cultural Psychiatry*. London: Academic Press.

Social Class

***Definition:* The term 'social class' has been used in a variety of ways in social science and remains contested. There is little doubt that all societies contain some people at the top who are rich and powerful and those at the bottom who are poor and powerless. The debates about social class then revolve around ways of defining and measuring differences in strata that exist between these extremes.**

Key points: • *Problems in defining social class are outlined* • *The relationship between social class and mental health problems is discussed, along with difficulties in interpreting the meaning of the relationship.*

Overall the relationship between social class and mental health is straightforward. The lower a person's social class position, the higher the probability of them being diagnosed with a mental health problem. However, this broad generalization contains contradictions and uncertainties, which are discussed below. Before that it should be noted that social class remains contested within social science. Social stratification is defined within these debates by various combinations of labour market position, socio-economic status, prestige, educational level, rank and property.

A relevant shift in Western European societies in the last 50 years has been from a pyramid structure of class to one of a diamond. The peak of both remains the same (the minority who are very rich and powerful). However, there has been a reduction in blue collar work, the traditional notion of manual working class people working in manufacturing industries, and an enlargement of white collar labour in service industries. The latter does not imply high levels of earning. Moreover, many in the service sector are in insecure employment. At the base of the new diamond is a group sometimes called the 'underclass', or what Marx and Engels called the 'lumpenproletariat'. These are people who are unemployed and often unemployable. They represent a social class which is reproduced, in a stable fashion, over several generations. They are chronically outside the labour market, poorly educated, living in poverty and susceptible to a range of social problems including substance abuse, mental health problems and criminality.

SOCIAL CLASS PREDICTS DIAGNOSIS

The overall correlation between social class and mental health – the class gradient of an inverse relationship between class position and prevalence of mental health problems – contains exceptions. Some diagnoses occur less frequently in lower class groups. These include eating disorders and obsessive-compulsive personality disorder. However, these are exceptions that prove the rule. The prevalence of those diagnosed with anxiety states, depression, anti-social personality disorder and schizophrenia (between them the most common diagnoses made in specialist mental health services) is significantly higher in the poorest stratum of society. The section on Cause and Constructs also points out that labour market disadvantage is important but not straightforward. The chronically unemployed are less distressed than those who are poorly employed (in stressful, poorly paid and insecure jobs). Single marital status is also a good predictor of mental health problems. As with class itself the question then begged is whether the disadvantage of single status is a product or cause of mental health problems, which leads to the next point.

THE DIRECTION OF CAUSALITY REMAINS UNCERTAIN

A problem for psychiatric epidemiology is that it only maps cases not causes. This is because for the functional diagnoses, causes are unknown or in dispute. Consequently, two antagonistic hypotheses have arisen, when a correlation is found between the prevalence of a diagnosis and a social variable. The first assumes that social stress causes mental health problems. The second assumes that inherited or acquired causes of mental health problems lead to the patient being socially disadvantaged. In the first case, high prevalence rates in the lower classes are taken to indicate the particular stressors associated with poverty. In the second case, it is assumed that the patient's illness leads to a downward 'social drift'. Usually the term 'social selection' hypothesis is used to connote this idea about social drift. A common intermediate position is the 'stress–vulnerability' hypothesis, which contends that patients susceptible to developing mental health problems may be buffered from this outcome by protective benign social conditions or precipitated into a mental health problem by adverse conditions. It is certainly the case that, in all social classes, people have a mixture of stressful events and buffering or protective experiences. However, the richer and more powerful a person is the more likely it is that the ratio of the two favours the protective experiences. A further complication here is that each of the three hypotheses may be more likely for some problems than others. For example, post-traumatic stress disorder is fairly well predicted by external stressors. Emergency service workers and battered wives have high prevalence rates of PTSD. In the case of the 'common cold' of psychiatry, 'depression', higher rates are found in the unemployed. However, not all acutely stressed people develop PTSD and not all unemployed people are depressed. This point suggests that individual differences exist about vulnerability within the same social circumstances. At the same time, diagnoses favoured for the social selection hypotheses, such as 'schizophrenia' do not follow neat genetic rules. Here the converse argument applies: why is it that some people but not others become psychotic in those with a genetic loading? It is probable that the peculiar stressors affecting vulnerable individuals trigger a mental health problem. These cautions, about the interpretation of the interaction between social stress and individual vulnerability, indicate that any particular diagnostic outcome is likely to have multi-factorial antecedents or aetiological pathways.

THE RELEVANCE OF THE UNCERTAIN DIRECTION OF CAUSALITY

Much of the argument about direction of causality is linked to the ideological investment of the protagonists. It matters to those on the political left that there is an evidence base for the health-sapping effects of poverty and social disadvantage. Evidence for the social stress hypothesis is also evidence for the need for social justice. Equally, it matters to those on the political right that poverty and social disadvantage can be accounted for by the behaviour or biology of their inhabitants. Genetic faults or fecklessness in the poor can be used to justify a natural order of inequality. Leaving aside these ideological preferences, the personal consequences of having a mental health problem become an over-riding consideration of patients (rather than the causes). This point is discussed further in the sections on Causes and Constructs and on Stigma and Social Exclusion. If the direction of primary causes remains in question, this is not the case for the relapse and maintenance of problems. In other words, a consequence of being stigmatized, socially excluded and living in poor conditions is that people with pre-existing mental health problems are made vulnerable to relapse and find recovery extra difficult, compared to those who are better off and more powerful.

See also: *causes and constructs; social exclusion; stigma; psychiatric epidemiology; race.*

FURTHER READING

Dohrenwend, B.P. (1990) 'Socioeconomic status (SES) and psychiatric disorders: are the issues still compelling?', *Social Psychiatry and Psychiatric Epidemiology*, 25: 4–47.

Eaton, W.W. and Muntaner, C. (1999) 'Socioeconomic stratification and mental disorder', in A.V. Horwitz and T.L. Scheid (eds), *A Handbook for the Study of Mental Health*. Cambridge: Cambridge University Press.

Eaton, W.W., Anthony, J., Gallo, J., Cai, G., Tien, A., Romanoski, A., Lyketsos, C. and Chen L-S. (1997) 'Natural history of DIS/DSM major depression: the Baltimore follow up', *Archives of General Psychiatry*, 54: 993–9.

Rogers, A. and Pilgrim, D. (2003) *Mental Health and Inequality*. Basingstoke: Palgrave.

Race

***Definition:* Race is controversial to define. Genetic distinctions between groups of humans (other than based on sex) have little empirical basis. Racial distinctions arose from anthropological investigations carried out by colonial powers and reflected the social categorizations of colonized indigenous people. However, because of colonization, the social identity of these people became real for them and others.**

Key points: *• Case studies of Afro-Caribbean and Irish people are provided to illustrate the relationship between race and mental health in a British post-colonial context • Implication for understanding racial differences in mental health are discussed.*

As the above definition indicates, race is scientifically dubious but socially real. For example, people of African origin dispersed by the slave trade throughout the Americas and economic migration later in Europe, now willingly call themselves 'black'. The relevance of this general socio-political point is that the health, including mental health, of previously colonized or enslaved people can be studied. When this happens, we find that it is the shared post-colonial context, which predicts differences in mental health status, not particular physical characteristics such as skin colour. This is illustrated in the British post-colonial context by examining the mental health of Afro-Caribbean and Irish people (Rogers and Pilgrim, 2005).

THE MENTAL HEALTH OF AFRO-CARIBBEAN PEOPLE

The term Afro-Caribbean (increasingly shifting to 'African-Caribbean') refers to black people who either still live in the Caribbean or who have moved to Britain. The term is now also used to describe their British-born children and grand-children ('British-born blacks'). Britain is an ex-colonial power, which enslaved and forcibly transported African people.

Afro-Caribbean people have higher rates of diagnosis for schizophrenia but lower rates for depression and suicide than indigenous whites (Cochrane, 1977). Young males are particularly likely to be diagnosed as psychotic. Higher rates of cannabis use in this group and their style of public behaviour, which is out of sync with indigenous white culture, have been mooted as contributory factors in this picture. The cultural gap, about norms of behaviour and the problems of intelligibility this creates, is discussed by Littlewood and Lipsedge (1997). Young male Afro-Caribbeans are particularly over-represented in secure provision and on locked wards (Fernando et al., 1998; Mohan et al., 1997). An unresolved debate about over-representation is whether it is actual (black and Irish people are mad more often) or whether it is a function of misdiagnosis (Sashidharan, 1993). The hypotheses are of course not mutually exclusive. Reviewing the competing hypotheses of raised prevalence rates of diagnosed schizophrenia in Afro-Caribbeans, Jablensky (1999) concluded that 'the causes of the Afro-Caribbean phenomenon remain obscure'.

THE MENTAL HEALTH OF IRISH PEOPLE

The data on Irish people highlight why the stresses of racism, based purely on skin colour, are not an adequate explanation of differences in mental health status (Bracken et al., 1998; Greenslade, 1992). Although Afro-Caribbean people (especially second generation young males) are vulnerable to psychosis, prevalence rates of all diagnostic categories are higher than for the indigenous (non-Irish) whites in Britain. Both Irish women and men are over-represented in psychiatric populations. They are twice as likely to be admitted to inpatient units as Afro-Caribbeans and three times more likely to be admitted than their English white counterparts (Cochrane and Bal, 1989). A variety of hypotheses about the over-representation of the Irish in psychiatric statistics addressing child-rearing practices, alienation from an imposed English ruling class culture, the over-bearing and sexually repressive nature of the Catholic Church and the confusions of a post-colonial identity can be found in the literature (Kenny, 1985; O'Mahony and Delanty, 1998; Scheper-Hughes, 1979).

IMPLICATIONS

What are the implications of comparing and contrasting these two ex-colonized groups for our understanding of the relationship between race and mental health?

The first point to emphasize is that given the white skin of the Irish, racism based on skin colour may be a stressor but is not one that accounts for racial differences in mental health. A confirmation of this is that young Asian men are not over-represented in psychiatric populations but young Afro-Caribbean men are (Cochrane and Bal, 1989).

A second point is that while both groups are post-colonial remnants of forced migration, the circumstances for each were different. The Irish were not enslaved but starved and dispossessed by British landlords. Africans lost or adapted their languages when they encountered English. In Ireland, Gaelic was suppressed – a trend of the English colonizers on the Celtic fringe throughout the British Isles.

Third, the circumstances of migration to Great Britain were similar in some ways but not others. Employment opportunities governed population movement in each. However, it was a continuous flow from the proximate Ireland over two centuries but only for prescribed limited periods for those from the Caribbean. During the 1950s and 1960s, they both encountered hateful notices in rental housing such as, 'No blacks. No Irish. No dogs'. Both were poor groups in unskilled or semi-skilled work. While the West Indian immigrants came to a perceived 'motherland', the island of Ireland was under continued British occupation and fought an unresolved war of independence with its colonizing neighbour. Migrants criss-crossing the Irish Sea embodied this tension. These histories of slavery and starvation, and the alienation it created in both, culturally resonated down the generations of each group.

Fourth, as ex-colonized people, Afro-Caribbeans and the Irish have been recurrently stigmatized and rejected. For those born in Britain they have nowhere to 'return to'. As a consequence, the mental health system, as an extension of the apparatus of coercive control of the State, is a repository for internal banishment. It is a place of segregation for those whose 'origin, sentiment or citizenship assigns them elsewhere' (Gilroy, 1987). A confirmation of this point is that these groups are also over-represented in the prison population, not just in involuntary specialist mental health services.

Fifth, and following from the previous point, whatever the causal explanations for over-representation, the racial bias means that these groups are disproportionately dealt with by specialist mental health services. As the latter are dominated by coercion, this outcome can be thought of as a form of structural disadvantage for these groups.

See also: *segregation; cross-cultural psychiatry; eugenics.*

REFERENCES

Bracken, P.J., Greenslade, L., Griffen, B. and Smyth, M. (1998) 'Mental health and ethnicity: an Irish dimension', *British Journal of Psychiatry*, 172: 103–5.

Cochrane, R. (1977) 'Mental illness in immigrants to England and Wales: an analysis of mental hospital admissions, 1971', *Social Psychiatry*, 12: 2–35.

Cochrane, R. and Bal, S. (1989) 'Mental hospital admission rates of immigrants to England: a comparison of 1971 and 1981', *Social Psychiatry*, 24: 2–11.

Fernando, S., Ndegwa, D. and Wilson, M. (1998) *Forensic Psychiatry, Race and Culture*. London: Routledge.

Gilroy, P. (1987) *There Ain't No Black in the Union Jack*. London: Hutchinson.

Greenslade, L. (1992) 'White skin, white masks: psychological distress among the Irish in Britain', in P. O'Sullivan (ed.), *The Irish in the New Communities*. Leicester: Leicester University Press.

Jablensky, A. (1999) 'Schizophrenia: epidemiology', *Current Opinion in Psychiatry*, 12: 19–28.

Kenny, V. (1985) 'The post-colonial personality', *Crane Bag*, 9: 70–8.

Littlewood, R. and Lipsedge, M. (1997) *Aliens and Alienists: Ethnic Minorities and Psychiatry*. Harmondsworth: Penguin.

Mohan, D., Murray, K., Taylor, P. and Stead, P. (1997) 'Developments in the use of regional secure unit beds over a 12-year period', *Journal of Forensic Psychiatry*, 2: 321–35.

O'Mahony, P. and Delanty, G. (1998) *Rethinking Irish History: Nationalism, Identity and Ideology*. Basingstoke: Macmillan.

Rogers, A. and Pilgrim, D. (2005) *A Sociology of Mental Health and Illness (Third Edition)*. Maidenhead: Open University Press.

Sashidharan, S.P. (1993) 'Afro-Caribbeans and schizophrenia: the ethnic vulnerability hypothesis re-examined', *International Review of Psychiatry*, 5: 129–44.

Scheper-Hughes, N. (1979) *Saints, Scholars and Schizophrenics*. Berkeley, CA: University of California Press.

Gender

***Definition:* Gender refers to descriptions of the role division of girls and boys and men and women in society. Sex refers to descriptions of a division based on biological features of the internal and external genitalia. Gender is a social description and sex is a biological one. In practice, often the two terms are used interchangeably in the professional literature.**

Key points: • *The complex relationship between gender and mental health is outlined* • *Factors accounting for the relationship are discussed.*

The relationship between gender and mental health is complex and it contains a core contradiction. On the one hand, generally women are more likely to receive a psychiatric diagnosis though, as will be noted later, this claim is sometimes contested. On the other (and this claim is certain), men are more likely to be treated coercively within specialist mental health services. The key phrase here is 'more likely'. With the inevitable exception of diagnoses linked to female physiology, such as 'premenstrual tension' and 'premenstrual syndrome', men and women may receive any diagnosis. And although secure mental health services are overwhelmingly populated by male patients, women can be found in them. While they are in a minority in secure services, women tend to be more vulnerable to abuse in them than are men.

Most of the over-representation calculated for women is accounted for by particular diagnoses (especially depression, panic disorder, agoraphobia, borderline personality disorder and eating disorders) (Gelder et al., 2001; Lepine and Lellouch, 1995). Most of the male over-representation in secure services is reflected in, and arises from, the higher prevalence of anti-social personality disorder (or psychopathic disorder in British law) and the management of some sex offenders within mental health facilities. The great majority of sex offenders are men. Sex differences are not apparent across the life span in relation to the diagnosis of the functional psychoses but the dementias are more prevalent in women (because on average they live longer). There are some sex differences, though, within the life span in relation to the diagnosis of the functional psychoses.

The inclusion or exclusion of certain diagnoses, when comparing men and women, can make the difference in representation between the two groups appear to be significant or non-existent. Moreover, claims about female over-representation have only appeared since the Second World War – there is little evidence from before then that sex differences in diagnosis were present. Arguments prevail then about whether levels of representation are real or whether they reflect methodological artefacts (Busfield, 1982; Gove and Geerken, 1977; Nazroo, 1995).

A number of points can be developed about this complex picture.

- *Professional decision making may be gendered* Some feminists have argued that, from its inception, the profession of psychiatry has targeted female deviance (e.g. Chesler, 1972). Showalter (1987) argued that women were over-represented in the Victorian asylums. However, Busfield (1996) notes that a more careful look at the evidence for this claim reveals that Showalter's case is unfounded.

Women lived longer in the asylums so their numbers were greater. Busfield argues that female over-representation in the asylum system was thus an artefact of the life span and was not, as Showalter claims, evidence of a patriarchal psychiatric focus on female madness. There is some evidence that in primary care GPs are more likely to identify mental health problems in women than men (Barrett and Roberts, 1978; Goldberg and Huxley, 1980). This is not merely a matter of more frequent contact (see the next point) but it also seems to reflect sex stereotyping by medical practitioners;

- *Gender representation may reflect type of service contact* There is a strong case for arguing that much of the gender difference can be accounted for service contact differences and style of help seeking. Women consult GPs more frequently than men (Rickwood and Braithwaite, 1994). Also, when men do consult they are less disclosing about distress than women (Blaxter, 1990). As a consequence, diagnoses made in a voluntary context will be applied less often to men. Moreover, the high contact with primary care services has led to the excessive prescription of psychotropic drugs to women for neurotic distress (Gabe and Lipshitsz-Phillips, 1982). For this reason, iatrogenic addiction to prescribed medication is greater in women than men;
- *Academic and journalistic accounts may be gendered* There has been a tendency for the social scientific academic discourse to conflate gender with women (Cameron and Bernades, 1998). This has had the effect, at times, of skewing research interest in mental health, with the consequence that we know more about women's mental health than men's. A good example of this is the seminal study by Brown and Harris (1978) of women and depression. This began as a study of *social class* and depression in the community, with the original intention of studying male as well as female respondents. However, this gender-balanced aspiration was dropped because the researchers predicted that women were more likely to be at home to be interviewed than men. Another example of skewed interest is in relation to the consequences of higher levels of prescribed medication for women noted in the previous point. This has been associated with a portrayal in the mass media of women being weaker and more dependent than men because of their higher rate of addiction to prescribed drugs (Bury and Gabe, 1990);
- *Social stress may generate real sex differences in mental health* Gove (1984) argues that the differences in rates of diagnosis are mainly a function of differences in social stress. This is most evident in relation

to eating disorders and sexual victimization. In the former case social pressures about body image affect females more than males. In the latter case, women are more frequently victims of sex attacks than men. However, men are more frequently victims of physical assault from strangers. Domestic violence is often discussed in terms of singular female victimization. However, the evidence suggests that sex differences are actually small or even non-existent (in terms of reported rates of assaults) (Rogers and Pilgrim, 2003). But women are more seriously injured in violent incidents and are more likely to remain traumatized (Nazroo, 1995). Trauma leads to a range of post-traumatic symptoms including anxiety, depression and panic disorder. If trauma is gendered in society then this will translate into gendered mental health problems;

- *Mental health services are an extension of the State apparatus of social control* This point is fairly unambiguous in relation to male dangerousness. Men are over-represented in both prisons and secure mental health facilities. Generally, men are violent more often than women. As a consequence, men with mental health problems are violent more often than women with mental health problems and they are treated more restrictively within the mental health system, as they are elsewhere.

To summarize, when we try to account for gender differences in diagnosis, treatment and service contact a number of factors may be operating. Some of these are competing hypotheses. Some are not mutually exclusive. Also, the topic of gender exemplifies a tension between one explanatory approach, which focuses on constructs or the social negotiation of gendered mental health (e.g. the potential bias in professional decision-making and the skewed academic focus on women) and another based upon causal empirical claims of real differences. For example, because women suffer peculiar social stresses, live longer and contact health services more than men and in a different way, these real differences produce direct effects on the recorded incidence and prevalence of mental health problems. Gender differences probably represent the outcome of a mixture of real and socially constructed processes (Busfield, 1988). For now, though, the list provided above is not a formula for a strong consensus about this concluding point. It is more an arena of dispute.

See also: *causes and constructs; forensic mental health services; primary care; eating disorders; fear; sadness.*

REFERENCES

Barrett, M. and Roberts, H. (1978) 'Doctors and their patients', in H. Smart and B. Smart (eds), *Women, Sexuality and Social Control*. London: Routledge and Kegan Paul.
Blaxter, M. (1990) *Health and Lifestyles*. London: Routledge.
Brown, G. and Harris, T. (1978) *The Social Origins of Depression*. London: Tavistock.
Bury, M. and Gabe, J. (1990) 'Hooked? Media responses to tranquillizer dependence', in P. Abbott and G. Payne (eds), *New Directions in the Sociology of Health*. London: Falmer Press.
Busfield, J. (1982) 'Gender and mental illness', *International Journal of Mental Health*, 11 (12): 46–66.
Busfield, J. (1988) 'Mental illness as a social product or social construct: a contradiction in feminists' arguments?', *Sociology of Health and Illness*, 10: 521–42.
Busfield, J. (1996) *Men, Women and Madness: Understanding Gender and Mental Disorder*. London: Macmillan.
Cameron, E. and Bernades, J. (1998) 'Gender and disadvantage in health: men's health for a change', *Sociology of Health and Illness*, 20 (5): 673–93.
Chesler, P. (1972) *Women and Madness*. New York: Doubleday.
Gabe, J. and Lipshitz-Phillips, S. (1982) 'Evil necessity? The meaning of benzodiazepine use for women patients from one general practice', *Sociology of Health and Illness*, 4 (2): 201–11.
Gelder, M., Mayou, R. and Cowen, P. (2001) *Shorter Oxford Textbook of Psychiatry*. Oxford: Oxford University Press.
Goldberg, D. and Huxley, P. (1980) *Mental Illness in the Community*. London: Tavistock.
Gove, W. (1984) 'Gender differences in mental and physical illness: the effects of fixed and nurturant roles', *Social Science and Medicine*, 19 (2): 77–91.
Gove, W. and Geerken, M. (1977) 'Response bias in surveys of mental health: an empirical investigation', *American Journal of Sociology*, 82: 1289–317.
Lepine, J.P. and Lellouch, J. (1995) 'Diagnosis and epidemiology of agoraphobia and social phobia', *Clinical Neuropharmacology*, 18 (2): 15–26.
Nazroo, J.Y. (1995) 'Uncovering gender differences in the use of marital violence: the effect of methodology', *Sociology*, 29 (3): 475–9.
Nazroo, J.Y., Edwards, A.C. and Brown, G.W. (1998) 'Gender differences in the prevalence of depression: artefact, alternative disorders, biology or roles?', *Sociology of Health and Illness*, 20 (3): 3112–330.
Rickwood, D.J. and Braithwaite, V.A. (1994) 'Social psychological factors affecting help seeking for emotional problems', *Social Science and Medicine*, 39 (4): 563–72.
Rogers, A. and Pilgrim, D. (2003) *Mental Health and Inequality*. Basingstoke: Palgrave.
Showalter, E. (1987) *The Female Malady*. London: Virago.

Age and Mental Health

Definition: This entry refers to the relationship across the life span between chronological age and mental health status.

Age and Mental Health

> ***Key points:*** *• Childhood has been the focus of competing theories about the development of mental health problems • Childhood and older adulthood are times of particular vulnerability to mental health problems.*

The relationship between age and mental health has been considered important broadly for two reasons. First, the idea that childhood is a phase of life when mental abnormality is primarily generated has held the attention of many researchers and theorists. Second, a longitudinal map of the relationship between age and mental health status reveals socio-political features about the life span. This section will address both of these points.

THE ROLE OF CHILDHOOD IN THE GENESIS OF MENTAL HEALTH PROBLEMS

In the section on Causes and Constructs it was noted that explanations for mental health problems remain varied. Bio-determinism, especially if it focuses on genetic explanations, minimizes the role of the post-natal environment. However, although many psychiatrists are bio-determinists, it is common for them to emphasize the interaction of biological vulnerability and environmental stressors. The latters are distributed unevenly across populations and across the life span.

Psychological theories place more of an emphasis upon the location of these uneven stressors in childhood. This can be seen in both psychoanalysis, with its emphasis on the dynamics of family life being internalized into psychodynamics in the child, and behaviourism, with its emphasis on the conditioning of anxiety responses. A further ambiguity is that some psychological theories such as Kleinian psychoanalysis conceded that individual differences in the inheritance of aggression can alter the proneness of the developing child to develop forms of psychopathology. By contrast, other psychoanalytical writers such as Winnicott (1958) and Bowlby (1951) emphasize the direct impact in infancy of environmental insults. This branch of psychoanalysis is much closer to the view advanced by behaviourists. Social theories of mental abnormality also emphasize the role of vulnerability in childhood, although multi-factorial models such as that offered by Brown and Harris (1978) suggest that contemporary contextual factors, not just historical ones, are important.

DIFFERENCES IN MENTAL HEALTH ACROSS THE LIFE SPAN

Whatever the competing theories say about childhood, one thing that is not in doubt is that general measures of mental health seem to indicate that it is a difficult phase of life. Community studies suggest that between 11% and 26% of children manifest distress or dysfunction, though only 3% to 6% of under 16s receive the attention of specialist mental health services (Bird et al., 1988; Costello et al., 1988). According to these studies, the prevalence of mental health problems in children has increased in recent times. Dysfunctional children then go on to experience educational disadvantage. In turn this leads to labour market disadvantage in later life and an increased probability of criminal activity.

When the family environment of distressed or dysfunctional children is studied it is evident that they are subjected to high levels of neglect and abuse, with estimates ranging from 20% to 65% (Quinn and Epstein, 1998). These pathogenic families are also disproportionately poor, though because of the range of mental health problems in childhood and variations in the mediating role of family life, it is important not to see the link between poverty and distress as being direct and simple. Not only do many poor families produce psychologically robust children but many richer families do not. What is at issue here are statistical tendencies. Poverty increases the risk of mental health problems (throughout the life span) but does not singularly determine those problems.

One of the main stressors in childhood with good predictive value is sexual abuse. The main version of this is intra-familial abuse with step-fathers being more likely to be the abuser than biological fathers. Sexual abuse occurs in all social classes. Girls are more at risk of intra-familial abuse but boys are more likely to be abused by paedophiles from outside the family (Rogers and Pilgrim, 2003).

Childhood problems transfer into adulthood. Longitudinal studies looking at cohorts of children from birth to adulthood (e.g. the 1970 British Cohort Study and the 1958 National Child Development Study) demonstrate this abiding impact of early childhood difficulties. The interaction of social class position and existence of mental health problems become particularly relevant. These studies demonstrate that:

- The existence of psychological problems and lower paternal class in adolescence predicts enduring mental health problems in adulthood;
- Achieved social class in adulthood is also predicted by paternal class and the existence of psychological problems in adolescence;

- The continuation of psychological difficulties is greater for men than women;
- Women demonstrate more inter-generational social mobility than men.

During middle adulthood average mental health scores improve. This may seem surprising given the commonly assumed impact of the mid-life crisis. In fact across the life span mental health problems can be plotted as a U-shaped curve. The highest rates of mental health problems occur in children and in the very old (Wade and Cairney, 1997). In old age the biopsychosocial model finds its greatest fit. Older people encounter a number of interacting challenges to their mental health:

- The incidence and prevalence of dementia increase with age;
- However, twice as many people over 70 are depressed than are dementing;
- Depression in old age is a function of psychological factors, such as cumulative bereavement reactions, as peers die around survivors (Clayton, 1998);
- Depression is also a function of somato-psychological reactions to multiple illnesses. Ageing increases the chances of co-morbidity and the latter brings with it disability and pain. These experiences in turn are depressing. Only 3% of men and 20% of women referred to specialist mental health services in old age are physically well (Dover and McWilliam, 1992). Only one in five older medical inpatients recovers from depressed mood before they die (Cole and Bellevance, 1997);
- There are gender differences in ageing. Women live slightly longer than men and so the prevalence of dementia is greater in females. When men are widowed they cope less well than women losing their spouse (Clayton, 1998). For this reason the risk of suicidal behaviour increases in older men. So too does the risk of substance misuse. Alcohol abuse in older men increases the chances of both depressive episodes and of premature death from cirrhosis of the liver (Helsing et al., 1982);
- Social factors are also relevant to predicting mental health problems in older people. The direct impact of poverty is one factor. Another is the restricted access to close confiding relationships in older people as they lose intimacy when spouses and friends die. Also social networks are restricted by changes in mobility. Housebound older people can less readily access their friends and relatives compared to younger days. Social contact is a protective factor against depression in all age

groups and so limitations on such contact increase the risk of depression (Murphy, 1982). The chances of depression also increase with residential care (Blazer, 1994). A final social factor to consider is that of elder abuse. Older people are subjected to abuse sometimes by their informal or paid carers with estimates or prevalence rates of abuse ranging from 8% to 15% (Hydle, 1993). Paveza and colleagues (1992) found that 5.4% of relatives of people with dementia were violent to patients within one year of the diagnosis. However, the same study found that 15.8% of dementing patients were also violent suggesting the possibility of an aggressive spiral in the carer–cared for relationship.

See also: *physical health; class; causes and constructs.*

REFERENCES

Bird, H., Canino, G., Rubio-Stipec, M., Gould, M.S., Ribera, J.C., Sesman, M., Woodberry, M., Heutos-Goldman, S., Pagan, A., Sanchez-Lakey, A. and Moscosco, M. (1988) 'Estimates of the prevalence of childhood maladjustment in a community survey in Puerto Rico', *Archives of General Psychiatry*, 43: 1120–6.

Blazer, D.G. (1994) 'Epidemiology of late-life depression', in I.S. Schneider, C.F. Reynolds, B.D. Lebowitz and A.J. Friedhoff (eds), *Diagnosis and Treatment of Depression in Late Life*. Washington, DC: American Psychiatric Press.

Bowlby, J. (1951) *Maternal Care and Mental Health*. Geneva: World Health Organization.

Brown, G. and Harris, T. (1978) *Social Origins of Depression*. London: Tavistock.

Clayton, P.J. (1998) 'The model of distress: the bereavement reaction', in B.P. Dohrenwend (ed.), *Adversity, Stress and Psychopathology*. Oxford: Oxford University Press.

Cole, M.G. and Bellevance, F. (1997) 'Depression in elderly patients: a met-analysis of outcomes', *Canadian Medical Association Journal*, 157: 1055–60.

Costello, E.J., Edelbrook, C.S., Costello, A.J., Dulcan, M.K., Burns, B. and Brent, D. (1988) 'Psychiatric disorders in primary care: the new hidden morbidity', *Paediatrics*, 82: 415–23.

Dover, S. and McWilliam, C. (1992) 'Physical illness associated with depression in the elderly in community-based and hospital patients', *Psychiatric Bulletin*, 16: 612–13.

Helsing, K.J., Comstock, G.W. and Szklo, M. (1982) 'Causes of death in widowed populations', *American Journal of Epidemiology*, 116: 524–32.

Hydle, I. (1993) 'Abuse and neglect in the elderly – a Nordic perspective', *Scandinavian Journal of Social Science*, 21 (2): 126–8.

Murphy, E. (1982) 'Social origins of depression in old age', *British Journal of Psychiatry*, 141: 135–42.

Paveza, G.J., Cohen, J.G. and Esdorfer, C. (1992) 'Severe family violence and Alzhiemer's disease: prevalence and risk factors', *Gerontologist*, 32 (4): 493–7.

Rogers, A. and Pilgrim, D. (2003) *Mental Health and Inequality*. Basingstoke:Palgrave.

Quinn, K.P and Epstein, M.H. (1998) 'Characteristics of children, youth and families served by local interagency systems of care', in M.H. Epstein, K.Kutash and A.

Duchnowski (eds), *Outcomes for Children and Youth with Behavioural and Emotional Disorders*. Austin, TX: Pro-Ed.
Wade, T.J. and Cairney, J. (1997) 'Age and depression in a nationally representative sample of Canadians', *Canadian Journal of Public Health*, 88: 297–302.
Winnicott, D.W. (1958) *Collected Works*. London: Hogarth Press.

The Pharmaceutical Industry

***Definition:* The pharmaceutical industry is the generic term used to describe the activity of the drug companies, which research and market medication. Given the central role of the latter in psychiatric practice, the industry plays a central role in mental health work.**

Key points: *• Shifts in the salience of drug treatments are outlined • The role of the drug companies in maintaining the dominance of a bio-medical approach to treatment is discussed.*

The success of the pharmaceutical industry over the past 50 years has been intimately entwined with both changes, and custom and practice, in the medical profession. This point has been particularly applicable to the treatment of mental health problems for two reasons. First, although psychiatrists have certainly been eclectic (with some specializing in psychotherapy and a small number flirting with psychosurgery), the profession's treatment response has been overwhelmingly medicinal. Secondly, most mental health problems have been treated in primary care. GPs in the main have used drugs to treat 'mild to moderate' conditions, dominated by diagnoses of anxiety states and depression. For this reason, it is little surprising that the pharmaceutical industry has frequently targeted GPs when marketing psychotropic medication.

The symbiotic relationship between the medical profession and the drug companies can be thought of in three historical phases.

BEFORE THE 1950s – THE PRE-REVOLUTIONARY PHASE

It would be wrong to accuse the drug companies of being the primary determinant of the bio-medical emphasis in psychiatry. From the beginning, in the Victorian period, the psychiatric profession emphasized biological causation. The shell-shock problem of the First World War momentarily diverted attention from this trajectory, allowing psychological theory and practice into the mental health service arena. But, other than during periods of warfare, it was a question of 'business as usual' in asylum psychiatry. Prior to the 1950s, psychiatrists had only a few biological options to calm patients: bromides, barbiturates, paraldehyde, opiates and a few synthesized tranquillizers, such as scopolamine. As a result, a medicinal response to madness was augmented by psychosurgery, seclusion, shocks (electrically or chemically induced), wet packs and baths. During this phase the psychiatric profession tended to view drugs as one of a few options to combine to manage madness. They were not ascribed special curative powers. However, this was about to change.

THE 1950s – THE 'PHARMACOLOGICAL REVOLUTION'

After the Second World War, a number of drugs were introduced to treat mental health problems. For this reason, this period has been characterized as the 'pharmacological revolution'. This discourse of revolution was reflected in the aspirations claimed for drug treatments. It is at this point that terms like 'anti-psychotic' and 'anti-depressant' were coined. During the 1950s the pharmaceutical industry began to compete vigorously to synthesize and market a few types of drug in response to specific mental disorders. Lithium salts were introduced for mood disorders. The first anti-psychotic was introduced (chlorpromazine), as well as the first anxiolytic (minor tranquillizer) to treat anxiety states – the benzodiazepine, Librium. Two types of anti-depressants also appeared: the tricyclic drugs and the monoamine oxidase inhibitors.

AFTER THE 1950s – THE REVOLUTION POSTPONED?

Once the pattern of pharmacological optimism had been established, drugs began to dominate psychiatric practice. Some in the profession demonstrated that ward activity and psycho-social interventions were important components of treatment and rehabilitation. Others were to show that anti-psychotic and anti-depressant medication had their best impact if complemented by psychological interventions. All too often though, patients, whatever their diagnosis, were to find themselves being treated singularly with pills or injections. The reputation (but not the use) of drug treatments was to decline for a number of reasons.

Average dose levels of anti-psychotics began to rise, with the consequence that an international pandemic of iatrogenic movement disorders became evident. After the 1960s, psychotic patients were made obvious by their shuffling gait, twitching limbs and grimacing faces. In primary care a different iatrogenic problem emerged. The widespread use of the benzodiazepines as minor tranquillizers and sleeping pills meant that many patients had become addicted to drugs, which no longer had any therapeutic value for them. (The benefits of benzodiazepines wane after a couple of weeks.)

More iatrogenic problems were to follow. Because of high dose levels ('megadosing') and drug cocktails ('polypharmacy'), the anti-psychotics began to cause acute cardio-toxicity and sudden death in some patients. An irony here is that chlorpromazine was originally sold over the counter in oral form to prevent nausea and sickness. It only became a danger to life when it was administered by mental health professionals in injected form. Death rates also rose because of the poor control of the adverse movement disorder effects of anti-psychotics.

One particular minor tranquillizer was to create a widely reported iatrogenic tragedy. In the early 1960s, Contergan (thalidomide) was marketed widely to GPs. It soon became evident that its administration during pregnancy was to create congenital deformities. Before the drug was withdrawn over 6000 babies were born with severe physical abnormalities.

During the 1980s newer forms of anti-psychotic and anti-depressant agents were introduced, with claims to greater efficacy and fewer movement disorder effects than the older drugs, which had constituted the 'pharmacological revolution'. However, these were not without their problems. Some caused blood abnormalities and had to be monitored closely (clozaril). Others were deemed unsafe in clinical practice and were withdrawn because of their cardio-toxic effects (sertindole). The new anti-depressants became particularly controversial as it became evident that they were associated with raised rates of suicide and aggression in some patients.

Defenders of the continued central use of drugs for mental health problems point out that the risks that they create to patients have to be set against the benefits that accrue. For example, the newer anti-depressants may raise the chances of suicide, but the older ones were more toxic and so created more accidental deaths. Also, untreated depression itself increases the risk of suicide. Moreover, drugs are cost-effective because they are much cheaper to deploy than labour-intensive alternatives (such as counselling or family therapy).

Probably the biggest credibility problem the medical profession has in relation to drug treatments is their dominant role. User groups largely complain not of drug treatments *per se* but of their unimaginative use. Typically, if a drug is not working, the prescriber will raise the dose level, try another version of the same class or add another drug. Patients (and their relatives) will ask for talking treatments instead of, or as well as, drug treatments. These demands reflect poor supply in mental health service routines. Ironically, these reasonable expectations are consistent with the evidence that maximum therapeutic effects occur when treatment packages combine drugs and talking treatments.

Doctors are over-reliant on drug company information to guide their practice and their professional training emphasizes the prescription pad. Investment in psychological treatments is a low priority. Finally, the drug companies are highly enmeshed with the continued professional development of psychiatrists and GPs. They typically fund training events and use these as opportunities to promote new drugs and maintain a continued focus on a medicinal approach to mental health problems.

See also: *biological interventions; psychological interventions; segregation.*

FURTHER READING

Baldesserini, R.J. (1999) 'Psychopharmacology', in A.M. Nicholi (ed.), *The Harvard Guide to Psychiatry*. London: Harvard University Press.

Breggin, P. (1993) *Toxic Psychiatry*. London: Fontana.

Brown, P. and Funk, S.C. (1986) 'Tardive dyskinesia: barriers to the professional recognition of iatrogenic disease', *Journal of Health and Social Behaviour*, 27: 116–32.

Fisher, S. and Greenberg, R.P. (eds) (1997) *From Placebo to Panacea: Putting Psychiatric Drugs to the Test*. New York: Wiley.

Healy, D. (1997) *The Anti-depressant Era*. London: Harvester.

Klass, A. (1975) *There's Gold in Them Thar Pills*. Harmondsworth: Penguin.

Tyrer, P., Harrison-Read, P. and van Horn, E. (1997) *Drug Treatment in Psychiatry: A Guide for the Community Mental Health Worker*. Oxford: Butterworth/Heinemann.

Warfare

Definition: *'state of war, campaigning, being engaged in war . . .' (Concise English Dictionary)*

Key points: *• The impact of war on mental health policy and on psychiatric theory and practice is described • The governmental preoccupation with the dangerousness of patients is placed in the context of the scale of violence associated with modern warfare.*

This entry appears in a book on mental health for two main reasons. First, warfare has been an important determinant of shifts in mental health policy and professional theory and practice. Second, it provides a global backdrop of violence to judge patient dangerousness against.

THE IMPACT OF WAR ON POLICY, THEORY AND PRACTICE

By the end of the nineteenth century, the system of large asylums was defining the stable present and likely future of psychiatry. This institutional containment of madness, on behalf of civil society, was at the centre of this policy emphasis. All this was to change with the First World War.

The eugenic emphasis in the asylums transferred poorly to these new conditions. Working class volunteers and officers and gentleman ('England's finest blood') broke down with predictable regularity in the war of attrition between 1914 and 1918 (Stone, 1985). 'Shell-shock' (since, variously dubbed 'war neurosis', 'battle fatigue' or 'post-traumatic stress disorder') simply could not be accounted for within the eugenic framework preferred by the medical superintendents of the civilian asylums. This view was tantamount to treason, if applied to soldier patients who were not conscripts. An alternative view, offered by the 'shellshock' doctors, was that some form of interaction, between extreme external stress and inner psychological vulnerability, accounted for the symptoms evident in the casualties of the trenches (Salmon, 1917). These patients were not the assumed degenerates of the asylum system but decent, ordinary and, in civilian life, apparently mentally stable people, who had broken down under conditions of extreme adversity (Keane, 1998).

A psycho-social approach to mental disorder was thus made possible by the conditions of warfare. Moreover, the jurisdiction of psychiatry consequently shifted and expanded. Neurosis had been of little concern to the alienists and mad-doctors of the Victorian period. Conditions of warfare obliged all parties – psychiatrists, politicians, civil servants and the relatives of returning soldiers – to take another version of mental disorder seriously.

This wider view of the role of psychiatry in society influenced the first major British reform of mental health legislation since the 1890 Lunacy Act. The 1930 Mental Treatment Act introduced a voluntary status for some boarders in mental hospitals and indicated the beginnings of community care. By the time a second period of hostility with Germany was becoming evident by the late 1930s, the government did not call upon asylum doctors for advice. Instead, the legacy of the shell-shock doctors was rewarded by a psychoanalyst, J.R. Rees, being appointed as head of the Army Psychiatric Services in 1938.

The Second World War was to have two major impacts in subsequent decades. First, the inability of the military medical services to deal individually with a new generation of traumatized combatants between 1939 and 1945 led to experiments in group work. Both group psychotherapy and therapeutic communities were created in this wartime period in military hospitals. Their legacy was to shape post-war NHS psychotherapy.

Another major impact of the Second World War was the invention of the term 'institutional neurosis', which was also called 'institutionalism' or 'institutionalization'. (The last of these terms has proved to be confusing. In the literature it also describes the policy of mass segregation in the asylums.) The germ of the concept of institutional neurosis came from the visit of a medical student with the Red Cross to observe the opening of the concentration camps. Russell Barton (1958) watched as skeletal inmates in unsanitary conditions paced around with arms folded. When asked to move to more fresh and clean conditions by the liberating forces, the inmates refused. After the war, Barton noticed that psychiatric patients in the large asylums manifested similar stereotypical behaviour and an irrational dependency on the institution.

A final example of the impact of the Second World War occurred during the 1960s and 1970s in Italy. The shame of fascism and the sensitivities of warehousing devalued people out of sight and mind, given the post-war evidence of the labour and death camps, and led to a strong movement for desegregation. In 1978 Law 180 was passed to close all large mental hospitals in Italy. A resonance about the camps probably influenced (but did not solely determine) hospital run down and closure, throughout Western Europe.

WARFARE AS INSTITUTIONAL VIOLENCE

An irony of governmental preoccupation with people with mental health problems as a source of violence is one of scale. If all of the acts of violence committed by individuals, globally, in the last 100 years (whether or not they were considered to be mentally disordered) were added together, the total would pale into insignificance in the context of warfare. The latter has been responsible for the recurrent mass killing of swathes of the civilian population by the military wing of the State in many countries during the same period.

The problem with the use of terms such as 'First World War' and 'Second World War' is that they understate the unending nature of global warfare. For example, between 1945 and 1990 there were 150 wars leading to the deaths of 22 million people (Goldson, 1993). Since 1990 we have seen wars in the Balkans, the Middle East and in Africa, which have continued this trend of State sponsored mass killing. The pattern of modern warfare has been less and less about military casualties and more and more about the annihilation, persecution and traumatization of millions of unarmed civilians. The psychological consequences for survivors are now immeasurable, as they extend into subsequent generations (Solkoff, 1992).

Unlike the patients they are concerned to control, for fear of violence towards others, politicians are unconstrained in their decision making about embarking on or prolonging warfare. For from being distrusted or socially controlled for their dangerous actions, politicians in this context are often the beneficiaries of violence. They stand to gain (and occasionally lose) votes. Loss of their liberty is rarely an outcome for them.

See also: *mental health policy; risks to and from people with mental health problems; eugenics.*

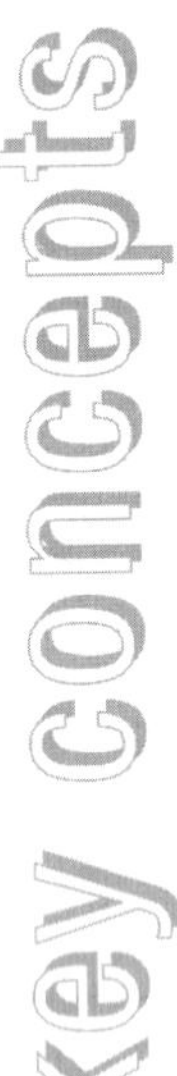

REFERENCES

Barton, W.R. (1958) *Institutional Neurosis*. Bristol: Wright and Sons.

Goldson, E. (1993) 'War is not good for children', in L.A. Leavitt and N.A. Fox (eds), *The Psychological Effects of War and Violence on Children*. Hillsdale, NJ: Erlbaum.

Keane, T.M. (1998) 'Psychological effects of human combat', in B.P. Dohrenwend (ed.), *Adversity, Stress and Psychopathology*. Oxford: Oxford University Press.

Salmon, T.W. (1917) 'The care and treatment of diseases and war neuroses: "shellshock" in the British army', *Mental Hygiene*, 1: 509–75.

Solkoff, N. (1992) 'Children of survivors of the holocaust: a critical review of the literature', *American Journal of Orthopsychiatry*, 62: 342–58.

Stone, M. (1985) 'Shellshock and the psychologists', in W.F. Bynum, R. Porter and M. Shepherd (eds), *The Anatomy of Madness (Volume II)*. London: Tavistock.